Child Health in a
Changing Society

BRITISH
PAEDIATRIC ASSOCIATION
1928–88

Child Health in a
Changing Society

EDITED BY

JOHN O. FORFAR

President, British Paediatric Association

OXFORD   NEW YORK   TOKYO
OXFORD UNIVERSITY PRESS
1988

Oxford University Press, Walton Street, Oxford OX2 6DP

Oxford New York Toronto
Delhi Bombay Calcutta Madras Karachi
Petaling Jaya Singapore Hong Kong Tokyo
Nairobi Dar es Salaam Cape Town
Melbourne Auckland
and associated companies in
Beirut Berlin Ibadan Nicosia

Oxford is a trade mark of Oxford University Press

British Library Cataloguing in Publication Data
Child health in changing society.
1. Paediatrics. 2. Child Health Services
I. Forfar, John O.   II. British Paediatric
Association
618.92   RJ45
ISBN 0-19-261687-0

Library of Congress Cataloging in Publication Data
Child health in a changing society.
At head of title: British Paediatric Association,
1928–88.
Includes bibliographies and index.
1. Pediatrics. 2. Child health services. I. Forfar,
John O. II. British Paediatric Association. [DNLM:
1. Child Health Services—Great Britain. 2. Pediatrics.
WA 320 C53457]
RJ47.C444   1988   362.1'9892   87-19619
ISBN 0-19-261687-0 (pbk.)

Processed by the Oxford Text System

Printed in Great Britain by
Biddles Ltd, Guildford and King's Lynn

Preface

Infancy and childhood are periods of particular hazard. They are times when many of the hereditary traits and disabilities handed down from earlier generations reveal themselves. The fragile infant at birth is subject to many physical and biochemical stresses and strains; the early months of life are a period of almost total dependence when the competence, care, and love of attendant parents, particularly the mother, are so essential; the adventurous toddler puts himself at particular risk of accidents and, as the range of his contacts widens, of infections derived from his playmates; schooling exposes the child with his immature personality to educational and psychological pressures which he may not be able to handle; adolescence creates problems of personality and identity and often social pressures to participate in unwholesome or dangerous activities which can damage health. Throughout infancy and childhood the continuous physical, psychological, and emotional changes resulting from growth and development create a vulnerability of their own.

Landor, the nineteenth century English poet, said,

Children are not men or women; they are almost as different creatures, in many respects, as if they never were to be the one or the other; they are as unlike as buds are unlike flowers, and almost as blossoms are unlike fruits.

Children are different and their health care presents many problems unique to their age group, but at the same time they *are* the buds and blossoms of life.

The possible blights and frosts of childhood disease are important determinants not only of health later in childhood but often also of health throughout adult life; and increasingly it is becoming recognized that lifestyle in childhood and adolescence may sow the seeds of a great deal of adult disability and disease.

Most parents are beset by recurring anxieties about their children. Organizations caring for children seek more information about child health. More widely throughout our society there runs a current of concern about the health and welfare of children, derived often from personal experience, preconceived ideas, the media, and conversational half-truths. In an age of mass communication there is a wider desire among the public to know more and more about child health issues. The background to child health is the ever changing physical, social, and economic environment to which the child is exposed.

This book seeks to present and discuss some current problems in child health and the influence on them of recent medical advances and the changing pattern of society. It seeks to do so in a manner appropriate for the interested layman and the child-care professional alike. Its authors are a number of members of the British Paediatric Association each contributing in an area of his or her own particular interest and expertise. Each contributor has been selected for his or her suitability to write on a particular topic.

The book is produced to mark the Diamond Jubilee of the British Paediatric Association (BPA), the professional organization for paediatricians in Britain.

The objectives of the BPA are to serve the public by advancing understanding of the origins, prevention, and treatment of disease in childhood, to further the study of child health and to promote excellence in paediatric practice. The responsibilities and activities of the Association include −

- providing authoritative views on childhood diseases
- promoting child health
- developing and promoting good practice in the care of sick, handicapped, disadvantaged, or deprived child
- promoting scientific research into the causes, prevention, and treatment of childhood disease
- disseminating the results of research through scientific meetings and the *Archives of Disease in Childhood,* the official journal of the Association
- acting as a national advisory body on all aspects of the health of children and adolescents, to government, the professions and voluntary and statutory bodies
- providing a national platform for paediatrics and child health
- providing representatives for international, national and local statutory committees dealing with childhood health and childhood disease

- maintaining an interest in and advising upon undergraduate, postgraduate, and continuing professional medical education in paediatrics and child health
- fostering good relations between British paediatricians and paediatricians in European and other overseas countries, including developing countries

The British Paediatric Association is a registered charity devoted to children: it is precluded from involving itself in matters such as the terms and conditions of service of its members.

It is hoped that this book will make a contribution to some of the objectives of the Association indicated above.

British Paediatric Association,   J.O.F
5 St. Andrews Place,
Regents Park,
London NW1 4LB

November 1987

Acknowledgements

All of those who have undertaken the task of writing for this book have done so as a contribution to the Diamond Jubilee of the British Paediatric Association. The Diamond Jubilee Working Party of the British Paediatric Association consisting of Professor J. D. Baum, Dr T. L. Chambers, Professor J. O. Forfar, Mrs Jean Gaffin, Sir Alan Reay, and Professor C. E. Stroud undertook the planning of the book.

Mrs Jean Gaffin and Dr Isobel Forfar read all of the text critically and made many valuable suggestions.

Thanks are due to those who kindly provided the photographs and gave permission for their reproduction; to the Department of Medical Illustration, Hospital for Sick Children, Great Ormond Street, London, for Plates I, III, IV, V, and XI; to the Department of Medical Illustration, St. James's Hospital, Leeds, for Plates II, VI, VII, and IX; to the Archives of Disease in Childhood for Plates II and IX; to Mr Len Cumming, Royal Hospital for Sick Children, Edinburgh for Plates VIII, X, XII, and XIII; and to Mr Tom McFetter, Simpson Memorial Maternity Pavilion, Royal Infirmary, Edinburgh, for Plates XIV, XV, and XVI.

Contents

Contributors

Professor Eva Alberman, MD, FRCP, FFCM, Professor of Clinical Epidemiology, London Hospital Medical College, Department of Clinical Epidemiology, Turner Street, London E2 2AD.

Professor J. D. Baum, MA, MSc, MD, FRCP, Professor of Child Health (Institute of Child Health), University of Bristol, Department of Child Health, Hospital for Sick Children, St Michael's Hill, Bristol BS2 8BJ.

Dr. Martin Bax, DM, MRCP, Senior Research Fellow, Community Paediatric Research Unit, Westminster Children's Hospital, Vincent Square, London SW1P 2NS.

Professor Martin Bobrow, DSc, MBChB, FRCP, MRCPath, Prince Philip Professor of Paediatric Research, United Medical and Dental Schools of Guy's and St Thomas's Hospital, University of London, Paediatric Research Unit, Guy's Hospital Tower, London Bridge, London SE1 9RT.

Professor A. G. M. Campbell, MB, ChB, FRCPE, DCH, Professor of Child Health, University of Aberdeen, Honorary Consultant Paediatrician, Grampian Health Board, Royal Aberdeen Children's Hospital, Foresterhill, Cornhill Road, Aberdeen AB9 2ZD.

Dr Richard W. I. Cooke, MD, FRCP, DCH, Reader in Child Health (Neonatal Medicine), University of Liverpool, Mersey Regional NICU, Liverpool Maternity Hospital, Liverpool L7 7BN.

Professor Donald Court, CBE, MD, FRCP, Hon.FCST, FRCGP, FRSM, Emeritus Professor of Child Health, University of Newcastle, 8 Towers Avenue, Jesmond, Newcastle upon Tyne NE2 3QE.

Dr Pamela A. Davies, MD, FRCP, DCH, Lately Honorary Consultant Paediatrician, Hammersmith Hospital, and Reader in Paediatrics, Institute of Child Health, London, 103c Clarendon Road, London W11 4JG.

Professor John O. Forfar, MC, BSc, MD, FRCP, FRCPE, FRCPG, FRSE, DCH, FACN, President, British Paediatric Association, Professor Emeritus of Child Life and Health, University of Edinburgh, 110 Ravelston Dykes, Edinburgh EH12 6HB.

Dr. Ann Gath, DM, FRCPsych, DCH, Consultant Child Psychiatrist, West Suffolk Hospital, Drummond Clinic, 21a Hill Road, Bury St Edmunds, Suffolk IP33 3PP.

Dr. Jean Golding, MA, PhD, Wellcome Senior Lecturer in Paediatric and Perinatal Epidemiology, Department of Child Health, University of Bristol, 77 St Michael's Hill, Bristol BS8 2BJ.

Professor David Hull, BSc, MBChB, FRCP, DObstRCOG, DCH, Professor of Child Health, University of Nottingham, Department of Child Health, University Hospital, Queen's Medical Centre, Nottingham NG7 2UH.

Dr. Aidan Macfarlane, MA, MBBChir, FRCP, Consultant Paediatrician (Child Health), Oxford District Health Authority, and Clinical Lecturer in Paediatrics, University of Oxford, Community Health Offices, Radcliffe Infirmary, Woodstock Road, Oxford.

Professor Roy Meadow, MA, FRCP, DObstRCOG, DCH, Professor of Paediatrics and Child Health, University of Leeds, and Honorary Consultant Paediatrician, St James's University Hospital, Leeds, Dept. of Paediatrics and Child Health, St James's University Hospital, Leeds LS9 7TF.

Professor Ross Mitchell, MD, FRCPE, DCH, Professor Emeritus of Child Health, University of Dundee, Craigard, Abertay Gardens, Barnhill, Dundee DD5 2SQ.

Professor Roger J. Robinson, MA, DPhil, BM, FRCP, Ferdinand James de Rothschild Professor of Paediatrics, United Medical and Dental Schools of Guy's and St Thomas's Hospitals, Dept. of Paediatrics, Guy's Hospital, London Bridge, London SE1 9RT.

Professor Michael Rutter, CBE, MD, FRCP, FRCPsych, FRS, Professor of Child Psychiatry and Honorary Director, MRC Child Psychiatry Unit, Institute of Physchiatry, Maudsley Hospital, Denmark Hill, London SE5 8AZ.

1

Worlds apart

DONALD COURT and EVA ALBERMAN

A changing society

The intention of this chapter is to examine the changing patterns over almost a century of health and disease in British children. The 60 years to the British Paediatric Association's (BPA's) jubilee year, 1988, have been claimed as a time in which the health of British children has improved to a greater degree than at any time in our history. Can this claim be justified, and can it be explained? Before we attempt to answer these questions we shall consider the meaning of the words we use. Health is well-being in its widest sense; disease is deviation, in differing degrees and various ways, from that optimum state. Our objective for every child is optimum well-being. Paediatricians and the BPA aim to contribute towards this through the provision of the medical care of, and the promotion of health in, the dependent, growing, developing and maturing child within his family and neighbourhood.

News from the front

We begin at the beginning of the century. Britain is at war. The military front is in South Africa, the health front in the recruiting offices at home. Between 40 and 60 per cent of men coming to enlist are found to be unfit for service. This alarming discovery prompted an examination of older schoolchildren, and many of them were found to be undernourished and suffering from recurring illness to an extent that rendered them unable to benefit from the education provided. This was no passing episode. Throughout the previous century of pomp and circumstance there was a continuing indifference to the health of children. Families were large, and high mortality among children was accepted as inevitable.

The following account gives the view of a paediatrician from an out-patient clinic in London at the turn of the century:

The first thing that struck me was the evidence of widespread poverty. Children were often ill-clad, dirty, malodorous and verminous. Undernourished children were common, and the diseases of malnutrition, such as rickets, were present in flagrant form. Anaemia was prevalent. Dried milk had not been invented, and diluted cows milk or condensed milk were the staple substitutes for breast milk. 'Tube bottles' were the rule, and what foul smelling contraptions they were. Almost every baby had its comforter, and with the low standard of hygiene it is not surprising that recurrent diarrhoea was the common sequel (Robert Hutchison 1940).

Almost a century later, after two world wars, Britain has been at peace for over forty years, but an uneasy peace beneath the clouds of a nuclear age. What news of her children now?

On every playing field and beach, and in every gymnasium and swimming-pool, the astonishing change can be seen. The majority of children are taller, better nourished, more robust, better educated, freer from disease, and on family occasions attractively dressed. They appear 'the picture of health' and, when compared with their ancestors 60 years before, 'worlds apart'. Such a change should be celebrated, without forgetting the children in our inner cities where poverty and hopelessness hold them and prevent them from sharing in the well-being of their neighbours who live in more favourable circumstances.

From death to life

Health can only be measured in the living. Today it is easier to plan the spacing and number of desired children, and when pregnant a woman expects to be conducted safely and courteously through pregnancy and to give birth to a live and undamaged baby. Survival through childhood is almost taken for granted. For the majority that expectation will come true, and Fig. 1.1 (for males only) shows how expectation of life from birth, age one year, and age fifteen years has increased over this century.

However, until recently the picture presented by vital statistics has been overshadowed by death. The habit of recording mortality rather than survival is firmly established.

Infant and childhood deaths

The contours of the graph in Fig. 1.2 tell their own story. Infant (first-year) mortality remained consistently high throughout the

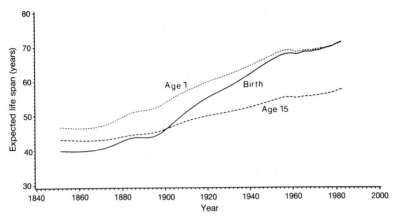

Fig. 1.1. Male life expectancies as at birth; age 1 year; and age 15 years. (*Annual Reports on Mortality Statistics, England and Wales: Series DH1.* Office of Population, Censuses and Surveys)

nineteenth century. From the beginning of the twentieth century a fall began which has continued until 1984, at which time a figure of 9.3 per thousand live births was reached, less than one-tenth the level at the turn of the century. Similar but less dramatic falls are seen for childhood mortality also.

Figure 1.3 illustrates more clearly the patterns of childhood and adolescent deaths from 1841 to 1980. Until very recently the four years after infancy (infancy = the first year of life) were the most hazardous, but within the last decade the rates have converged, with the lowest death rate being between the ages of 5 and 14. The rate between 15 and 19 years has flattened out. Over the period shown the overall picture is one of marked improvement, the general fall being interrupted only between 1916 and 1920, a time of war and of an influenza pandemic.

The reasons for these overall falls and trends in specific diseases will be examined in detail in order to provide guidance for our future policy and for those countries with current levels of mortality comparable to ours at the turn of the century.

The fall in infant mortality is one of the most spectacular advances in health in this or any other period in history. Why has it happened? Not through a corresponding rise in technical care of the new-born infant or of the infant during the first year of life. Chemotherapy and antibiotics, which have played an increasingly

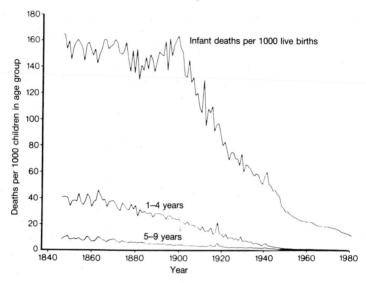

Fig. 1.2. Mortality rates at various ages per 1000 children in different age groups (1846–1981) (Macfarlane and Mugford 1984, Fig. 3.1b).

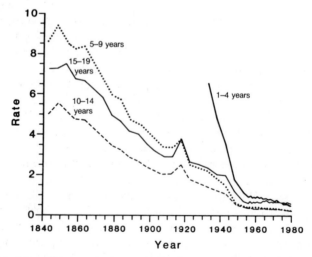

Fig. 1.3. Mortality rates in various age groups per 1000 population (1841–1980) (*Annual Reports on Mortality Statistics, England and Wales: Series DH1 No. 15.* Office of Population, Censuses and Surveys)

effective part in the second half of the century, were not available until 1936 and 1946, respectively. If the influences responsible were not particular they must, at least in the early phase, have been general. What changes were taking place in our culture which could so powerfully affect the infant in the womb and in the first year of life?

In the century leading up to the Great Exhibition of 1851 Britain had become the industrial leader of the world and, by the end of the century which followed, her 'standard of living' had doubled. Such a change produces its effects by the interaction within society of many processes, resulting in high employment, higher wages, better housing, more varied food and a rising standard of formal and popular education. While we still do not fully understand all the pathways which link standard of living with health, it is clear that consequent improvements in nutrition, the reduction of high infection rates associated with overcrowding, and the improved knowledge and expectations of health care are all important factors. Moreover the improved health of infants carries over into their adult life, which in turn enhances reproductive success and the health of the next generation.

Improvements, in medical and nursing care, such as the training of paediatricians and paediatric nurses, began in a specific way in centres such as Edinburgh in 1931, but did not undergo more general expansion until after 1945 when a steady development of university departments of Child Health and Paediatrics took place. A major professional contribution was the intensive study of the physiology and pathology of the fetus and of the new-born and the growing child. As the nature of these was elucidated rational care for the normal, the low birth-weight, and the morbid infant became possible. Much more intensive study of childhood diseases and of the methods of preventing and curing them, better nursing care and earlier treatment following the establishment of the National Health Service all played their part.

Within this framework of social improvement and new understanding many fruitful advances were to follow, including the development of special care units for the low birth-weight infant, better infant feeding, properly staffed and equipped hospital paediatric departments, the critical use of antibiotics and other specific and effective medications, a more effective school health service, and specialization within paediatrics. With the increased knowledge of the physiology of infants and children came a more detailed study of their respiratory and cardiac physiology and their biochemistry. This formed the basis of many newer therapeutic techniques and extended the age range of surgery in the young child down to the first weeks of life. The processes which have brought about this notable fall in infant mortality can thus be seen as a beneficial interaction between social improvement, physiological and pathological insight, and the rational care and treatment of childhood disease.

We cannot, however, enjoy the celebration of increasing survival and leave it there. National incidence hides local variations, and this is shown in Fig. 1.4. This is not a matter of geography but of economics. The figure for each region reflects relative poverty, the level of unemployment, and the ability or inability of a region to sustain long established industries or to replace them. These local differences are more strikingly revealed as the locality studied is smaller in size. If specific action is to follow this kind of analysis the electoral ward is a useful area to concentrate on, and there have now been numerous analyses demonstrating the close relationship between, particularly, infant mortality and local indices of deprivation.

Growth and development

The fall in infant and childhood mortality is not an isolated phenomenon, but a reflection of the remarkable changes in childhood growth and development which have accompanied changes in standards of living. It is unfortunate that despite numerous exhortations to the effect that a regular and permanent anthropometric surveillance of the British population should be instituted, none was instituted until recent decades. Nevertheless, what data exist point clearly to a substantial and consistent increase in the stature of British children over the last century. This is also true of other countries in which similar data have been collected.

This overall picture of increased growth in childhood conceals wide and systematic variations between groups of children with different living standards. These differences express, as clearly as any other data, the persisting gulf between different groups in our society. This is illustrated in Fig. 1.5, which gives an example of the downward deviation from the overall mean of the height of

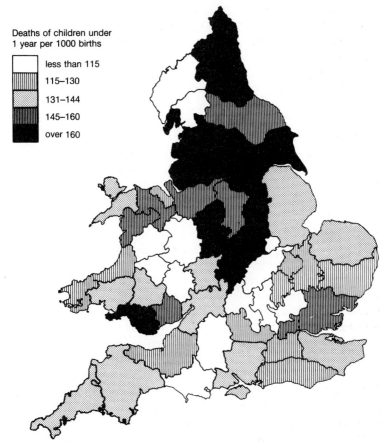

Deaths of children under
1 year per 1000 births

less than 115
115–130
131–144
145–160
over 160

Fig. 1.4. Infant deaths per 1000 live births in England and Wales (1976–80). (Macfarlane and Mugford 1984, Fig 3.12).

English children of fathers in manual and non-manual occupations with increasing numbers of siblings.

The changes in weight of children have been even more marked than the changes in height, and data from two of the national cohort studies (studies conducted over a period of years of children born at the same time) confirm that obesity in childhood may be becoming a new health hazard. Certainly there have been major changes in average weight for height, the full significance of which is still doubtful.

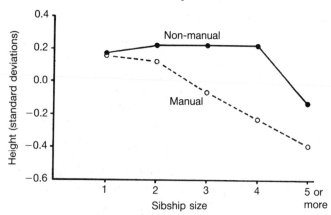

Fig. 1.5. Heights of children in England expressed in standard deviation score (SDS) according to the occupational status of their fathers and sibship size. (From Rona, R. J., Swan, A. V., and Altman, D. G. (1978). *Journal of Epidemiology and Community Health.* **32**, 147–54.)

It cannot however be in question that the improved nutritional status of our children, however measured, has been accompanied by a remarkable fall in vulnerability to disease. This can be demonstrated, on a population basis, both directly—the prevalence of respiratory symptoms being negatively related to the height of primary school children—and indirectly, the rapid fall in the prevalence of diseases such as tuberculosis, and the plummeting case fatality of such disease as measles and whooping cough, being almost certainly, due to the improved health of children secondary to their nutritional status.

Associated with the increases in growth and weight has been a reduction in the age of onset of puberty, which has brought with it a revolution in sexual behaviour in adolescence for which, inexplicably, we were not prepared. Early sexual maturity, an increase in permissiveness, easy access to alcohol, tobacco, drugs, fast cars, and sexually transmitted diseases have together contributed considerably to the current problems of our adolescent children, problems that are replacing tuberculosis as a scourge of young adults.

However, none of these can totally detract from the achievements leading to the notable falls in childhood deaths which we have seen over the past 60 years.

The progressive mastery of diseases

Some of the specific diseases which, by their reduction in incidence, have caused the momentous changes in child mortality are set out in Table 1.1. Our forefathers would have been astonished at the elimination or control of the common fevers, which they regarded as one of the inescapable burdens of childhood.

There are some general and some specific reasons for these impressive falls in mortality over the last 75 years. As already mentioned, the general reasons are related to childrens' improved nutrition and to better housing without overcrowding; the particular processes will be dealt with as we condsider each individual disease.

The common fevers

Apart from tuberculosis the major scourges in the form of specific infectious diseases were those laid out in Table 1.1, which gives the *mortality* rates per million children between one and 14 years certified as due to these infections. Almost certainly related infections were included; diphtheria deaths probably included some deaths from acute laryngo-tracheo-bronchitis ('croup'), and whooping cough some deaths from other respiratory disease, but whatever the pathology the death-rate had fallen to low levels even before immunization had been introduced, except in the case of diphtheria where the sharp fall in mortality after the war years can be attributed mainly to large-scale immunization.

In so far as *morbidity* is concerned, the numbers of our children suffering from these unpleasant and still often dangerous diseases remains unacceptably high (Figs. 1.6 and 1.7). As recently as 1982 the number of children in England and Wales notified as having measles was 94 195, and whooping cough 65 810, and because many cases go unnoticed these represent only a proportion of those suffering from these illnesses. These children are the victims of our voluntary system of immunization, with parents often unresponsive to the call for measles immunization, possibly because of a mistaken idea that this is a mild, uncomplicated disease, and to whooping cough protection because of the fear of vaccine complication. The effect on morbidity of the fall in the uptake of vaccination consequent to this fear is shown clearly in Fig. 1.7.

Another dreaded infectious disease, poliomyelitis, has been virtually eliminated by a very effective vaccine given by mouth. The

Table 1.1

Deaths of children aged 1–14 years from various causes. Adapted and updated from Court (1976, Table 2, p. 41)

Cause	1911–15		1931–35		1956–60		1970–74		1976–80	
	No	Rate/mill	No	Rate/mill	No	Rate/mill	No	Rate/mill	No	Rate/mill
Diphtheria	23 380	447	13 820	311	15	0	1	0	0	0
Measles	48 986	936	10 874	254	210	4	111	2	83	1.6
Whooping cough	20 182	385	6071	137	72	1	7	0	10	0.2
Gastro-enteritis	25 560	488	3485	78	447	9	487	9	137	2.7
Tuberculosis	46 459	887	14 544	327	306	6	71	1	35	0.7
Scarlet fever	9901	189	2589	58	7	0	0	0	–	–
Rheumatic fever*	3495	67	2465	55	139	3	6	0	35	0.7
Cancer	2388	46	2853	64	3971	83	3743	69	2931	57.3
Pneumonia and bronchitis	76 643	1464	28 226	635	3347	70	2330	43	1454	28.4
Accidents	18 500	353	12 126	273	6736	140	7214	133	5273	103.0

* The figures are not strictly comparable because of revision of the ICD (International Classification of Disease) Code.

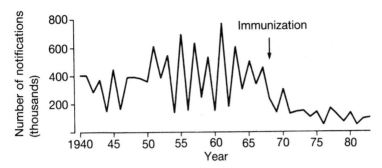

Fig. 1.6. Measles notification in England and Wales (1940–83). (From *Annual Reviews of Communicable Disease* (1983). PHLS, Communicable Disease Centre, and Office of Population, Censuses and Surveys.)

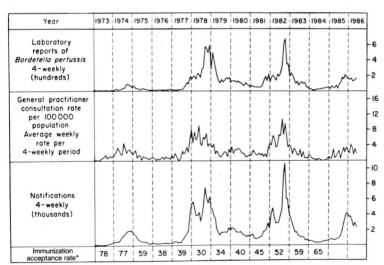

*Percentage of children completing vaccination by the end of the second calendar year after birth.

Fig. 1.7. Whooping cough: England and Wales (1973–86) (*Communicable Disease Report*, Weekly Edition 86/87).

prevention of paralysis, which often led to widespread handicap and death, is a notable example of the mastery of disease in this century.

Specific vaccination plays a part in the prevention of a wider range of illness. Tetanus, though infrequent, is extremely difficult to treat, but tetanus toxoid will prevent the disease. Rubella (German measles) is a mild disease, but is dangerous for the fetus, damaging the brain, sight, and hearing, if contracted by the mother early in pregnancy. This unpleasant syndrome is slowly being reduced by giving rubella vaccine to girls aged 11 to 13 years; it could probably be eliminated if parents, general practitioners, and school doctors made certain that every girl received the vaccine at the right age.

Gastro-enteritis

An infectious disease which used to dominate the hotter periods of the year was epidemic gastro-enteritis or summer diarrhoea. At the beginning of the century, in 1911–1915, it caused 25 000 deaths in children aged one to 15 years, a figure which had fallen to less than 150 in 1976–1980. Three factors brought about this change. The first was the social effects of improved housing and sanitation, better disposal of refuse, greater freedom from dust on public thoroughfares, and better storage and preparation of food. The second factor was the increase in knowledge about the causal bacteria and viruses, although much remains to be learnt about these. The third factor was the estimation of the state of dehydration, and the giving of water and salt in sufficient quantities and at the correct rate to restore the disordered physiology to normal. The introduction of simple methods of oral hydration on a worldwide basis and particularly in developing countries has probably been one of the most important advances of the last decade, and owes much to the research work and the advocacy of members of the British Paediatric Association.

Tuberculosis

Perhaps the mastery of illness which would have impressed our ancestors most would be the control of tuberculosis in children. Tuberculosis is an infectious illness caught from an adult or adolescent with tuberculous lung disease. It is curable and pre-ventable. The first step in control is to know what can happen in the child once the organism (mycobacterium tuberculosis) has entered the body. It lodges in the lungs, the pharynx, the bowel, and at times the skin, and forms an area of necrosis or breakdown of tissue from which the mycobacteria travel to the related lymph glands. Soon a variety of responses follow, of which the main one is lymphatic or blood-stream spread. The latter can give rise to tuberculous meningitis, which, before present management became available, was uniformly fatal. Following the blood-stream spread small inflammatory foci can develop in many organs, especially the lungs, kidneys, and bones. These manifestations of primary tuberculosis may heal or remain, only to break down in adolescence or adult life, giving rise to the progressive disease we know as pulmonary or adult tuberculosis. Understanding the difference between the response of the body to first and later contact with the mycobacterium is an important key to control and eradication.

A comparable series of events occurred when infected milk was widespread, untreated, and readily available for drinking. Since the heat treatment (pasteurisation) of all milk became established this intestinal form of tuberculosis has almost disappeared. The danger is from holidays on outlying farms where one of the pleasures is to be given 'milk straight from the cow'.

An important element in the control of tuberculosis was the discovery of a number of drugs effective against the disease, of which the best combination is paramino-salycylic acid (PAS) and isoniazid (INH), with streptomycin for tuberculous meningitis.

The measures which will achieve control and eradication of tuberculosis are not always clearly understood. In addition to the pasteurization of milk these comprise the reduction of infective reservoirs by the recognition and treatment of all cases of infective pulmonary tuberculosis, the prevention of primary infection by the use of BCG vaccine, and, where relevant, the treatment of primary infection in children whether this is associated with clinical illness or not.

The control of tuberculosis has been described in detail because all the processes by which childhood disease can be prevented and cured come together in this disease. The importance of good nutrition in reducing vulnerability is recognized; the use of a vaccine (BCG) prevents the development of a natural infection; and when that infection occurs there is an effective range of chemotherapeutic and antibiotic agents for eradication and cure. This continuing process requires from the health service an organization which will make sure that every child's tuberculosis state is known, and that every child who has been in contact with adult tuberculosis receives surveillance and, if necessary, treatment.

Scarlet fever and rheumatic fever

There are two related diseases to be mentioned to complete our review of the mastery, or coincident fall, of certain childhood illnesses in this century.

The first is scarlet fever, which results from infection with a specific bacterium, the streptococcus. In the nineteenth century there were several cycles of severe streptococcal infection. From the beginning of this century these have steadily lost their lethal capacity, and scarlet fever today is a mild disease. In this instance the disappearance of severe illness and death over the century would seem to be independent of social change and due mainly to a decline in the virulence of the causal organism, the haemolytic streptococcus, which is its cause. Why this has happened we do not know.

The natural history of rheumatic fever, a disease usually resulting from a particular type of reaction to a streptococcal infection, has also changed completely. Although the incidence of rheumatic fever started to decline in the 1890s, it was still a major problem among children in the 1930s and 1940s with its residue of cardiac damage. However, in the late 1940s and early 1950s its occurrence rapidly declined, possibly due to better overall health of children, and less overcrowding, as well as to changes in the virulence of the streptococcus and the advent of antibiotics. The decline of rheumatic fever, which is now an extremely rare disease, did however begin before the widespread use of antibiotics for sore throats.

Investigations into the other arthritic diseases in childhood became possible when it was found that these were characterized by the presence of identifiable chemicals and specific cell types. Thus has emerged a pattern of a number of different clinical rheumatic entities, some apparently more common in persons of certain genetic types (HLA groups). For instance, one type of juvenile arthritis which involves only one or two joints and often damage to certain parts of the eye is associated with the presence of specific antibodies and HLA types DR5 and DR8. Newer tests have allowed further differentiation of disorders of the skin or ligaments, whose marked rarity at one'time would seem strange in a paediatric rheumatology clinic of today. In other words, specific and separate disease types within broad categories can now be recognized and the changes in their incidence monitored. These changes relate not only to better diagnostic facilities, but to some extent to changes in the population and to an increase in the number of children particularly vulnerable to certain types of disease. Examples are systemic lupus erythematosus and its variants (diseases affecting blood vessels and connective tissue and involving many organs in the body), particularly among the Asian communities.

Better diagnostic facilities and therefore better understanding of these diseases have allowed improved assessment of prognosis so that appropriate management can be applied early in the course of the disease. Moreover, with the increasing application of new scientific methods such as those of molecular biology to these diseases we can anticipate that by the end of the century the causation of many which are currently ill-understood will be revealed.

Increasing hope

There are also a number of other conditions, considered below, in which no means of primary prevention have yet been developed. The reasons for increasing hope that they will be controlled lies in better understanding of the nature of the disorders and in more rational and therefore more effective treatment. The diseases we use to illustrate this category cover many conditions needing surgical as well as medical care, including infection of the urinary tract, some forms of cancer, especially acute childhood leukaemia, and respiratory disease.

Infections of the urinary tract

The natural history of acute pyelonephritis (infection of the kidney) was described in the 1920s. The start is insidious, without symptoms, although bacteria are present in the urine, and it progresses to the fever and distress of an acute inflammation of the kidneys. This disorder is still a common, recurrent condition which can begin in infancy. It does its damage silently and is therefore a condition which must be looked for. The damage is to the substance of the kidney, which is progressively destroyed, but only if the circumstances are such that there is an obstruction in the urinary tract causing the infected urine to be pushed backwards.

After years of debate, certain things are clear. The slow wasting of the kidneys as a result of infection is a preventable cause of kidney failure and high blood pressure. At first it seemed necessary to correct the reflux of urine, if necessary by surgical means. Later it became evident that the danger came from the infection; if the initial attack of this, hopefully discovered near its beginning, is treated effectively, and recurrence prevented with continuing medication until the danger period is passed, the outlook is good.

Some forms of cancer

Cancer is the main disease preoccupation of our age, and is no longer a forbidden word. Many remember the darkness which surrounded discussion of the disease in children in the 1930s. When the diagnosis was made there was little further the physicians could do. Then in 1942 came the bizarre news from the USA that nitrogen mustard, a product developed in the First World War as a lethal gas, was effective against certain types of cancer of the lymph glands known as lymphoma and lymphosarcoma.

Up until then surgery and radiotherapy had been used in treatment, but the clinical use of nitrogen mustard reported in 1946 marked the beginning of chemotherapy in the treatment of cancer. By 1949 the second effective drug, aminopterin, came from the USA, and since then a variety of drugs capable of suppressing the metabolic function of certain cancer cells have been developed.

The next decade was a distressing time for children, parents, and paediatricians as the latter struggled to discover the effective dosage and necessary duration of treatment with these new drugs. The ulceration of the mouth, the loss of hair, and the wretchedness of the child, which were the unfortunate concomitants of treatment with these drugs, could only be endured. Yet parents, however distressed, never asked for the treatment to be stopped; they realized that they and the paediatrician were held together by a common bond of suffering and hope. 'If you think it can do any good, please go on' was the repeated plea. The patience and endurance of many parents and children has been largely rewarded.

For the last 20 years the search has continued for the best combination of surgery, radiotherapy, and chemotherapy. The advances have been stepwise rather than breakthroughs, but the really important step has been the systematic testing of drug régimes on a national scale both in Britain and the USA. 60 per cent of children developing acute lymphatic leukaemia now survive ten years or more, and some appear to be cured. These trials have necessitated the increasing centralization of treatment in special regional centres in which outcome is consistently improving. A more recent advance is bone marrow transplantation which may cure a small selected group of children with the rarer acute myeloid leukaemia.

We have thus moved a long way from the 1950s when all that could be offered for the child with leukaemia was support and palliative treatment without hope of a long-term survival. Now, for virtually all affected children, there is something that can be done with a real hope of cure. The overall survival for cancer in childhood is now over 60 per cent. Recent five-year survival curves for different cancers are shown in Fig. 1.8.

What next in the future treatment of childhood cancer? A change in the philosophy of care from 'cure at any cost' to 'cure at the least cost' is one change which economic factors are now imposing. There can still be a better deployment of the available treatments. The basic need however is for a better understanding of the cellular processes which we call 'cancer'. Here again molecular biology may come to our aid. Viruses cause leukaemia in animals, and at least one tumour in humans. Burkitt's lymphoma (a childhood tumour found widely throughout Africa) and a small group of adult leukaemias involving a particular lymph gland cell are known to be due to the Epstein–Barr virus. There are sufficient pointers here to examine further the role of viruses in the causation of at least some other cancers.

Respiratory infection

This is the main infective problem in childhood in our country today. In the family studies conducted in Newcastle, over the first five years of life, of every ten illnesses eight were infective: five of the eight were respiratory infections, and one of the five was bronchitis, bronchiolitis, or pneumonia. Deaths due to these infections have fallen from 76 000 in 1911–1915 to just under 1500 in 1976–1980, but mortality is no longer an effective measure of their effect on children. Parents beseech paediatricians to do

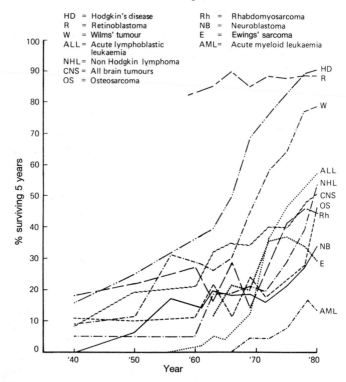

Fig. 1.8. Percentage of children surviving 5 years from the diagnosis of childhood cancer (1940–80) (A. W. Graff, The Children's Cancer Research Group, Oxford).

something about the repeated colds and coughs and sore throats which dominate so many children's early years. Fortunately the natural history of these disorders, especially those of the upper respiratory tract, shows a decline from age eight years onwards.

The greatest advance in our understanding of these respiratory infections that has occurred this century has been the progressive discovery of the respiratory viruses. In 1932 the virus of influenza A was discovered, but even 20 years later a cause for respiratory infections in children could only be found in 3 per cent of cases. By 1965 the respiratory syncytial virus, the most important virus in acute bronchiolitis of young infants, was identified, the para-influenza viruses were found to be associated with 'croup', and the adenovirus causing a range of illnesses including pneumonia had been isolated. Studies performed in the USA suggested that viruses were causally related to between 60 and 80 per cent of acute severe respiratory disease in children.

The next advance was the rapid identification of viruses by the use of immuno-fluorescent microscopy, thus allowing decisions on treatment to be made quickly.

The third discovery was the significance of the social dimension in these illnesses, as in others. Using the five social classes based on occupation of the father—from professional and managerial to unskilled—the Newcastle studies found an incidence of bronchitis, bronchiolitis, and pneumonia ten-times as great in Social Class V as in Social Class I. These findings have been replicated in many other studies since, and improvements in standard of living and housing are probably the most effective primary preventive measures we have.

Unfortunately, a continuing obstacle to management is that antiviral agents are so far only available for influenza A and Herpes virus hominis (the virus of primary herpetic stomatitis and of the 'cold sore') and these play a marginal role in children's respiratory infections. In spite of the success of the vaccines for measles, poliomyelitis and German measles, no comparable vaccines have been developed for the respiratory viruses except for influenza A. This makes it essential in treatment to look not only at the virus but at the disturbed physiology in the ill child. Here the major danger is that the respiratory disease temporarily interferes with oxygenation, but this can usually be remedied by modern methods of respiratory support.

Asthma

Another respiratory disorder—described by Hippocrates—is asthma. The advances in the last 25 years are these. First, long-term studies have shown the mechanism in these patients to be a too ready contraction of the smaller air passages due to their increased lability. This gives rise to episodic or continuing shortness of breath and the characteristic wheeze. This understanding has led to certain advances in treatment designed to prevent the abnormal contraction of the air passages—especially the use of certain bronchodilator drugs given by inhalation and the unexpected discovery that sodium cromoglycate, when taken regularly, again by inhalation, has a preventive effect. Unfortunately some of the bronchodilator drugs may have dangerous side-effects if used to excess, and the dilemma of management is to diagnose all children who can benefit from treatment whilst avoiding a dangerous overtreatment of the severe cases.

The persisting shadows

Here we include causes of impairment like accidents and dental decay where methods of primary prevention are well recognized but fail to be implemented, and those in which we still have much to learn, such as sudden unexpected infant death and problems of prematurity, epilepsy, diabetes, and child abuse.

Accidents

Accidents are now by far the most frequent cause of death in children between their first and fifteenth birthdays (Table 1.1). Although their number had been falling slowly the figure in Britain in 1984 was still 865. The circumstances in which they occurred included: on the road, 428; in the home, 204; burns, 83; and drowning, 58. They led to some two million children, i.e. one in six, attending Accident and Emergency Departments, with 133 000 being admitted to hospital. Many injuries were severe and, if the children survived, some would be permanently disabled.

Why, for so long, has a major cause of child death and disability aroused so little concern on the part of the public and those involved in professional care? Organizations have long existed with a commitment to accident prevention. One of the main reasons is related to the welfare of children as a whole. In this country children are lower on the scale of social priorities than in comparable countries, especially Sweden, the Netherlands, and Japan. We have yet to see children as full citizens whatever their age and wherever they live.

Thus in 1954, Sweden, prompted by her paediatricians, began to implement a national policy for the prevention of childhood accidents. In the next 30 years a significant fall in the number of deaths and disabilities occurred. The essence of the Swedish approach was the recognition of the developmental difference between the dependent yet growing child, the adventurous adolescent, and the established adult.

A conference in Newcastle-upon-Tyne in 1976 brought the Child Accident Prevention Committee (now the Child Accident Prevention Trust) into existence. Its methods have been to study each type of accident, the circumstances in which it occurred, the services available for treatment, and the measures necessary for prevention. A central conviction, shared with Sweden, is that a principal cause of childhood accidents is the material environment constructed by adults for adults. The Trust has brought to light unrecognized factors in each type of accident, seeking them out with the working assistance of the public, architects, builders, glass manufacturers, car designers, and the relevant departments of government—a necessary preliminary for rational forms of prevention. The causes have been found to be complex, each requiring a specific form of remedy.

If the first requirement and conviction regarding the prevention of accidents concerns the need to change the material environment, the second is the understanding that the growing child will have different accidents at different ages and that this must be taken into account in planning. In this country we have as yet seen little acceleration in the fall in the figures for death and disability due to accidents, but the Swedish experience that this is possible, gives hope.

Dental health

Dental decay is still prevalent in our society, and children are more susceptible than adults.

In 1927 studies on the dental health of London schoolchildren showed that at the age of five years more than 95 per cent had tooth decay. This state of affairs with involvement of both deciduous and permanent teeth continued until 1970. At this stage a number of surveys suggested that dental caries was declining. The extent and rate of this fall was measured nationally in 1973 and 1983 and over the ten years decay had diminished by one-third. At five years of age the proportion of teeth with some decay had fallen from 71 to 48 per cent, and at fifteen years the average number of teeth with evidence of decay had fallen from 8.4 to 5.6 per person. This improvement was related to several factors. The central advance was an emphasis on conservative dentistry. This resulted, for instance, in a fall in the need for a general anaesthetic during dental treatment in eight-year-old children from 49 to 27 per cent.

These figures are both encouraging and discouraging: encouraging because the incidence of decay is falling; discouraging because so much delay is occurring in preventing a preventable disease. If decay is preventable why is it not being prevented? There is one measure, the addition of fluoride to the water supply where the natural level is low, which would prevent a great deal of caries without relying on personal discipline. At present only 8 per cent of the people in Britain live in homes receiving water treated in this way, although many more would benefit from it. If caries was a lethal disease fluoridation would have been mandatory from the 1960s onwards. The procedure is safe and cheap, and now that the legal obstacles have gone water authorities are likely to extend fluoridation considerably. Even partial measures, fluoride in tooth-paste and the topical application of fluoride, have proved partly effective, although they only reach a proportion of children.

The next ten years should show a further fall in the incidence of tooth decay. This will provide the time and incentive to deal with early gum disorders which at present affect over half of our children and which are a major cause of tooth loss in adults.

Sudden unexpected deaths (*cot deaths*)

With the rapid fall in the number of deaths of infants and young children due to well recognized causes, sudden unexpected death is becoming increasingly important. This usually occurs in infants after the third month of life, but sometimes happens in the early part of the second year of life. Since 1971 such deaths have been identified on death certificates, and now account for about 1200 deaths a year in Britain, with one-third of these deaths occurring between four weeks and one year of age. Although in approximately half of these cases intensive investigations reveal a presumptive pathological cause, something like one in a thousand infants currently dies suddenly and unexpectedly without an identifiable pathological cause. This is not a new problem, and until fairly recently similar deaths were described as 'cot deaths' or ascribed to overlaying. The risk is higher and arises later in prematurely delivered infants, and may be related to the physiological developmental changes in breathing patterns which normally occur in the third month. Certainly this is an area of current concern to the public and to professionals alike.

Often confused with these truly unexplained deaths are those of infants who are known to have been ill, but whose deaths were nevertheless totally unexpected by their parents and often by the professionals caring for them. The risk of this latter category is least where there is a low threshold for parental and professional concern and where the organization of the child health services is optimal so that rapid and appropriate care is available even for apparently minor illnesses. A child health service needs to recognize the need for *early* assessment of childhood illness.

Problems of prematurity

Pre-term delivery (before the thirty-seventh week of pregnancy) remains as common as it was 60 years ago, but understanding of how to handle the pre-term baby has been transformed. We have relearnt the importance of adequate warmth. We have learnt something of the value of supplemental oxygen as well as its dangers for the premature brain and eye. We have discovered that babies deal with some drugs more slowly than adults, and that the pharmacology of drugs administered to them requires to be individually explored. Our understanding of the pre-term baby's nutritional needs has also increased. We are more aware of the important, subtle immunological properties of human breast milk. At the same time we know that it is difficult for breast milk to offer the baby weighing just 1 kg the calcium phosphate needed for healthy growth. We understand more how the new-born kidney deals with water and salt, and that a pre-term baby may have skin so thin and respiration so rapid and accentuated that up to one-third of all the water received can be lost invisibly. The most important issue for the small pre-term baby is to establish breathing, and we have learnt that immature babies lack the substance (surfactant) which reduces the surface tension of the tiny compartments of the lungs and by so doing promotes normal respiration. We have found ways of encouraging its production. Artificial ventilation, monitoring of oxygen and carbon dioxide levels in the blood, and treating the infections these babies get have resulted in the chance of survival being notably increased.

We have also learnt that parents need to be involved with their tiny babies, no matter how sick (Plates X and XVI), so that when they go home they and their babies are already closely bonded and the parents not fearful of handling their infants.

Yet, for all the progress of the last 60 years, many unsolved issues remain which threaten the health of young babies. We remain ignorant of the cause of spontaneous placental separation. We can recognize intra-uterine growth retardation more readily than in the past, but we are still ignorant of many of the factors which cause it and of what can be done about them. We do not know what initiates premature labour or, once started, how to stop it. We still know little of how to anticipate or prevent antepartum or intrapartum infection of the fetus. Perhaps most disappointing of all, while joint obstetric-paediatric advances in the last 30 years have reduced dramatically the numbers of maternal, still birth, and neonatal deaths, the number of survivors with cerebral palsy or mental retardation is as great as ever.

The central problem of survival after premature birth is now the quality of life these children achieve (see Chapter 3).

Epilepsy

This disorder has been known from the beginning of Man's history. It was well described by Hippocrates in the latter half of the fifth century BC. He insisted that it was a disease due to natural causes like any other and not a punishment inflicted by the gods. Advances in understanding came with the discovery in 1928 of electrical brain waves which could be recorded by the electro-encephalogram. The waves in the epileptic child often showed different forms from those found in the normal person.

The variety of brain tracings obtained in different forms of seizure also confirmed the accepted clinical view that epilepsy was not a single condition with a single cause but a diverse group of disorders showing seizures as a clinical feature. Studies of defined communities give the incidence at different ages. In one such study conducted over a 15-year period the incidence in children under the age of 5 was 7.2 per cent and, between 5 and 15 years, one per cent. Altogether in this community seven per cent had had a seizure at some time in the first 15 years. Other studies broadly agree, which suggests that there are some 60 000 children with controlled or continuing seizures in England and Wales at the present time. Drugs to control seizures have been improved in their effectiveness, depending on their level being regularly monitored in the blood or saliva, yet more than 2000 years after the epilepsies were described they remain a major personal problem.

Diabetes mellitus

The great advance in this century in this condition was the discovery of insulin by Sir Frederick Banting in 1921. Before that, control had depended on severe food restrictions resulting in emaciation and an early death.

Advances in management have taken two directions: first, the discovery of a range of insulins giving more consistent control and a better understanding of desirable diets; and second the passing of general management from the hospital clinic to the parents and the child, leaving the role of the doctor and the trained nurse or health visitor to one of education and support. The more the family understands about the child's disorder the better will the control be. This is a general principle which applies to many chronic diseases of childhood.

With such a notable improvement in the quality of life why have we set diabetes among the persisting shadows? For four reasons: effective control calls for a high degree of family discipline; complications often persist which can lead to the blocking of small arteries in the eye, the kidneys, and the limbs, and are indicators for many of a shortened life and death in middle age; means of prevention are as yet little understood; and cohort studies suggest that the disease may be increasing in frequency and presenting more often before five years of age.

However, when diabetic boys and girls of good physique are seen at an 'outward bound school', the improvement in their growth and vigour with disciplined control of their disease is a reason for some satisfaction. With this is the hope that prevention, through transplanting active insulin-producing cells, will make more rapid progress than at present we can achieve.

Child abuse

As accidental injury moves into the circle of planned prevention, increasing evidence of non-accidental injury, child neglect, and abuse is compelling a reluctant public and medical profession to face its extent and extraordinary complexity. Nothing is more tragic than the death of or injury to a child at the hands of those who should protect him. The most distressing accounts reach the Press, whose reaction is to look for someone to condemn. The problem needs to be seen first in an historical context. Violence to children by parents and other guardians has been a fact of human society from the beginning. Thomas Coram, in the eighteenth century, created the Foundling Hospital because he was deeply distressed at the number of dead infants he saw in the gutters and refuse heaps of London, and the exploitation of children of six and seven years of age in the mills and mines of Victorian England was notorious.

The initial response of professionals was a failure to see, followed by denial. Then came the recognition of the individual examples of severe neglect, physical injury, and sexual abuse. The present turning towards the problem began in 1946 when radiologists, firstly in the USA, began to recognize that certain combinations of broken bones and collection of blood beneath the skull (subdural haematoma) must have been due to injury, almost certainly inflicted by an adult. In the late 1950s following an American study of 3000 such children the concept of the 'Battered Child Syndrome' emerged. Pioneer paediatricians in Britain in the 1960s began to recognize the problem more frequently, and this was followed in the 1970s by a collective approach which included the social services, the child and family psychiatrists, and, where death or serious injury had occurred, the police. It was now clear that the bizarre and often widespread injuries were due to the infliction of injury usually by wilfully destructive parents. In the earlier stages many such parents are frightened and confused and more accepting of help. Many are found also to be haunted by memories of injuries and abuse suffered in their own unhappy childhood. Contrary to our natural wishes W. H. Auden's observation is true:

> Those to whom evil is done
> Do evil in return.

As the problem was increasingly recognized, a multidisciplinary approach developed. The aim of this was to guide the social services which carried the main professional responsibility in designing a programme of help for the family. It had been clear from the beginning that, while the child must be protected against further injury, the parents needed disciplined help to restrain their violent feelings and then to grow out of them. In some instances this could be provided in special hostels and units admitting mother and child, or by the provision of neighbourhood support providing continuing contact. Such efforts are sometimes successful but, where they are not, the outcome for the child at risk can be tragic. Deciding on the best course of action for the benefit of the child involves difficult medical and social judgements, which by the very nature of the problem cannot always be correct. The preventive answer lies in raising the standard of care for all children from conception onwards.

In the early 1980s, when an ordered though incomplete approach to physical injury had been achieved, the much wider problem of sexual abuse began to be increasingly recognized. This problem too has been present throughout history. Its extent is unmeasured, but we know already that it is distressingly frequent. We know too that the adult is in most cases a member of the family or a family friend. This too has long historical roots, but at some point it has damaging effects on the child, the adult involved, and the family. This unhappy problem deeply challenges our standards of child care, and the professionals who care for children will have to face up to it.

Handicap and death

Even after the improvements we have chronicled we are still left with children with special needs, whether because of physical, mental, or behavioural problems. Major advances have been made, not the least of which are the understanding that not all impairments or disabilities need lead to serious handicap, and that certain, particularly psychiatric, handicaps can be a consequence of the individual's social framework or material surroundings. With physical disabilities we are increasingly making use of technological aids to overcome many of the disadvantages which the disabilities impose. There has been much heart-searching and rethinking regarding the best educational provision for those with special needs, and above all we are learning to listen more to the parents and the affected children themselves.

The past 60 years have been notable too for major strides in the understanding of the effects of institutionalization, both short- and long-term, and the need, even for the most impaired child, of a normal family life. Sociologists have taught us something of the effects of stigmatization on the disabled and their families, and we are learning that independence is a goal to be aimed at by all, no matter what their limitations. We have learnt too that grieving is

a necessary part of coming to terms with death or disability, that
doctors cannot distance themselves from this, and that professionals
need to share with parents the decisions that must be made.

The social and racial dimension

Social class differentials

The theme of inequalities of health and of variations in risk of
premature death with socio-economic status runs unchanged
through the history of paediatrics over the past 60 years. Child
poverty remains with us, even if less common and less severe than
in Dickensian times, but an important new element is its link with
minority groups, as determined by ethnic origin, or with deviant
family structure, as in the single-parent family. In 1976 a wide and
detailed account of child health in its social setting was given in
the Report of the Committee on Child Health Services (Court
Report 1976). The call of the Black Report (DHSS 1980) was that
the abolition of child poverty should be adopted as a national goal
for the 1980s. As of 1987 there is no evidence that this is a political
priority.

Apart from intuitive abhorrence of distress and ill-health in
children the British population has not yet learnt that adult health
is built on the foundations laid in intra-uterine life and childhood.
Evidence is mounting that the social class differences observed in
adult height attributable to differences in childhood nutrition and
health, are associated with differences in the risk of premature adult
death and morbidity, and that the groups with high infant mortality
are those with a high risk of cardiovascular disease in adult life.
Not to put children as a political priority is short-sighted in every
way, and the consequence serious and long standing.

Are we our brothers' keepers?

It must be admitted, however, that the inequalities seen within this
country almost pale into insignificance when compared with those
seen throughout the world. There are countries now where the
poverty and misery are infinitely worse than they were in Britain
at the turn of the century. These are other worlds indeed, and
worse now that they can be contrasted with Western affluence and
that we know so much more about the prevention and treatment

of disease. The BPA continues to contribute to the medical care of developing societies, and the description of kwashiorkor, nutritional surveillance, and the prevention of gastro-intestinal deaths are all subjects to which BPA members have made great contributions. Again, however, other political priorities frequently dwarf any efforts that can be made by the caring professions. A new spark of hope was seen recently when Bob Geldof raised the concern of nearly all of our young people, and perhaps too members of the older generation who had almost given up hope of changing the circumstances of the billions of starving children throughout the world.

'The end is where we start from' (T. S. Eliot)

In our concern for the intact survival of children we have not, up to recently, devoted ourselves to linking aspects of childhood physiological, metabolic, and behavioural patterns to adult health. Only in the last few decades has there been large-scale research looking at the relationship between childhood and adult health. This has been foreshadowed by the important cohort studies for which British paediatrics is rightly famed. However, we still know remarkably little about the lifelong tracking of blood pressure or blood cholesterol levels, and the factors which affect these; the laying down in blood vessels of the atherosclerotic plaques which cause myocardial infarction (coronary thrombosis) or the rate of loss of brain cells or of neurological or sensory function. We do not even fully understand the factors which affect adult obesity, or those which particularly predispose to psychological problems. We accept political expediencies which do not adequately discourage abuse of tobacco or alcohol early in life. On a national scale we know that the diet of many of our children is less than desirable. We remain indifferent to survey findings demonstrating that most school meals as currently offered are likely to lay the foundations of atherosclerotic disease, and we accept high levels of un-employment in early adult life when we strongly suspect this of being undesirable in terms of future mental health.

In the Jubilee year of the BPA we still have much work to do if we are to match the achievements of our predecessors in reducing acute disease. It is becoming increasingly clear that the practice of paediatrics and the promotion of child health with which the BPA

is involved are of critical importance in the health of the nation—
important not only for the health of the child but equally for the
health of the adult.

Acknowledgements

We gratefully acknowledge the contribution of many colleagues
who helped with this chapter.

References

Auden, W. H. 'September 1 1939' in *Another time*. Faber and Faber,
London.
Court, D. (1976). *Fit for the future. Report of the Committee on Child
Health Services*. HMSO, London.
Department of Health and Social Security (1980). Inequalities in health:
report of a research working group. London: DHSS.
Eliot, T. S. (1986). Little Gidding: *Four quartets*. Faber and Faber, London.

2

Heritable diseases and congenital abnormality—the prospect for prevention

DAVID BAUM and MARTIN BOBROW

Introduction

The ultimate goal of medicine in society is the prevention of disease. In the short term, however, the goals for the physician dealing with an individual afflicted by a disease are different and include the relief of symptoms, the treatment of the disorder, and an effort to achieve a complete physical and psychological cure.

In dealing with hereditary diseases, very few of which are amenable to curative treatment, the contrast between these two orientations in modern medicine is striking, particularly so when dealing with the fetus and new-born infant and the young parents who share the burden of their infant's disorder.

Conditions resulting from disordered early embryogenesis (the period of approximately two months post-conception during which the embryo is developing into a fetus) often present as morphological malformations (disorders of shape or form) at the time of birth, for which treatment is limited and cure impossible. Such developmental disorders frequently include irreversible abnormalities of many organs including the brain, resulting in physical and mental handicap.

Disorders originating later in gestation, after the period of major organogenesis (the later period of fetal development when organs have developed their structure but have not yet developed their full size or function) is complete, may still result in profound abnormalities of development but are generally more likely to be limited to an individual organ. In this sense the defects may be more limited and amenable to treatment although rarely capable of complete cure.

Congenital abnormalities are present in at least 3 per cent of all new-born babies (Kaback 1984): additionally, disorders not evident at birth but of a predominantly genetic aetiology will become manifest later in life. Some of these abnormalities are incompatible with an independent life for the baby after birth; the majority result in varying degrees of morbidity and shortening of life expectation.

Genetically determined disorders account for between 11 and 27 per cent of admissions to children's wards in this country (Emery and Rimoin 1983) and are a major factor in 50 per cent of children's deaths (Roberts, Shavez, and Court 1970; Emery and Rimoin 1983). These figures apply to developed industrialized societies. The perspective in developing and largely rural communities is likely to be different.

Before considering the strategies which may be adopted in trying to reduce this burden of incurable disease in our society it may be helpful to deal with some basic concepts and the associated technical vocabulary.

Basic concepts

Genetic

Genetic (inherited) disorders are those where the causation is predominantly due to changes in the chemistry of the genetic material, DNA (deoxyribonucleic acid), which may be passed from one generation to another. They are thus genetically determined before conception takes place. The primary action of genetic material (genes) is to control the synthesis of biological materials. An abnormal make-up of DNA will result in abnormal protein synthesis within cells. This can take many forms and result in trains of events which can cause a wide range of diseases.

Congenital

Congenital disorders are those present at birth. They may have a genetic (preconceptual) basis but the majority result from a mishap in the development of the embryo or fetus *in utero* (post-conceptual).

An example of a genetically determined congenital disorder is albinism in which the inability to synthesize the body pigment melanin results in a 'colourless' new-born baby due to the complete absence of pigment in the hair and iris. By contrast an example of a non-genetically determined (post-conceptual) congenital disorder resulting in major congenital abnormality is rubella embryopathy, in which a previously normal embryo, infected by the rubella virus acquired by the mother during her pregnancy and transmitted to her fetus, suffers a range of severe physical abnormalities (for example, of the heart or eyes) evident at birth.

The categorization of abnormalities as genetic or developmental may be less clear-cut when they are not overtly manifest at birth. Examples of abnormalities which may be delayed in manifesting themselves include: among genetic disorders, inborn errors of metabolism which are not revealed until an affected infant is challenged by the extra-uterine environment—for example, the normal dietary amino acid load in a baby born with phenylketonuria; and among non-genetic developmental disorders, structural abnormalities of the heart or kidneys the manifestations of which may be delayed for months or even years after birth. A significantly delayed genetically determined disorder not manifest at birth is Huntington's chorea in which a characteristic dementia only becomes evident in middle life.

From these examples, and others which we will discuss later, it is evident that there is an intricate interplay between genetic make-up and environmental factors in the origin of many serious disorders of childhood and later life. While the genetic predispositions present at birth, indeed from conception onwards, may not be evident at birth, technical developments, as we shall see, may in future allow their identification.

Familial

The term familial is purely a descriptive one. The occurrence of the same disorder in more than one member of the family (familial aggregation) may lead to a suspicion of a genetic causation for the disorder; it is, however, equally compatible with a shared environmental factor, be that an infectious agent, a toxin, or a component of diet.

Conversely, many inherited disorders appear with no prior family history. For example, two-thirds of cases of Duchenne muscular dystrophy (a disease causing progressive and ultimately fatal weakness of muscles) are sporadic. This may be because the affected child represents a newly arisen mutant gene (a mutant gene is one whose character changes, usually for the worse, in an individual and is then passed on to the next generation) in that family; alternatively, chance alone may have determined that cases had not arisen in the preceding generation or two. In the extreme, a dominant condition (one carrying a one-in-two chance of transmission) which prohibits reproduction would never be passed on and would never show familial aggregation. Thus Duchenne muscular dystrophy, because affected individuals rarely procreate, is a good example of a disease the frequency of which in the population is more or less maintained constant largely as a result of recurrent mutation. Sickle cell disease (a disorder of blood causing anaemia and painful 'crises') is an example of a disorder which allows the 'carrier' to reproduce. The condition, common in certain races, carries some biological advantage to the individual in resisting malaria. It is likely that all the sickle cell genes in existence today are derived from a very small number of ancestral mutation events. It follows that strategies for reducing the incidence of these two types of disease, Duchenne muscular dystrophy and sickle cell anaemia, are likely to be very different.

Congenital abnormalities may be subdivided into three groups: Mendelian single-gene disorders, multifactoral disorders, and chromosomal disorders.

Mendelian single-gene disorders   These result from abnormalities of the detailed make-up of the DNA which constitutes the gene. They show classical patterns of inheritance: autosomal dominant, autosomal recessive, or sex-linked. With an autosomal dominant disorder, a patient suffering from the disease has a one-in-two chance of passing it on to his or her offspring. With an autosomal recessive disorder neither parent is affected by the disease but each carries (is a carrier of) an abnormal or recessive gene which does not express itself because it is paired with a normal gene which fulfils the required function (genes are paired). The child of parents both of whom carry one recessive gene has a one-in-four chance that he will inherit two of these abnormal genes and thus suffer from the disorder. A sex-linked disorder is one which occurs only in males and is carried by females. A male affected by a sex-linked disorder such as haemophilia will have normal sons but all his daughters will be carriers. A female who is a haemophilia carrier has a one-in-two chance that each of her sons will be affected by the disease and a one-in-two chance that each of her daughters will be carriers.

Multifactorial disorders   This is a much more common but less well defined group of disorders believed to result from an interaction of several genes together with one or more environmental factors. It is likely that many of the common disorders of mankind will eventually be explained on this basis. Reasonably clear examples include such common diseases as diabetes, high blood pressure, and certain structural malformations such as the neural tube (the primitive structure from which the brain and spinal cord are developed) defects of which spina bifida (see pp. 56 and 86) is the commonest type.

Although the multifactorial aetiology (causation) of disease is useful in concept, it is of limited predictive and practical value. At our present level of understanding recurrence risks for these disorders must usually be predicted from empirical family studies rather than be calculated accurately on theoretical grounds.

Chromosomal disorders These result from defects in the number or structure of chromosomes. Chromosomes are strands of material, present in the nuclei of cells, which contain the genes. In the human, normal body cells contain 46 chromosomes and the sperms and ova 23. The union of male and female sex cells at conception restores the 46 pattern. Most chromosome disorders are related to disturbances of redistribution of chromosomes which occur during the formation of sperm and egg cells (e.g. Down's syndrome in which there are 47 chromosomes in each body cell as opposed to the normal 46). Chromosome disorders represent a disorder on a macro scale compared with single-gene disorders. They are seldom familial.

Gene probes

The use of recombinant DNA techniques, (a system which detects DNA abnormalities chemically and can be applied to the identification of abnormal genes) can produce 'gene probes' which can be used for the diagnosis of specific inherited disorders. In a few cases, notably sickle cell anaemia, the gene probe can test directly whether or not the specific site mutation (i.e. the abnormal gene) is present. More often, however, direct testing for gene site mutation is not yet possible and it is necessary to test DNA sites close to, but not identical with, the site of mutation to indicate the presence of the latter. The nature of these adjacent sites is such that they act as 'markers' on the chromosome carrying the affected gene.

Predictions arising from such linked markers can only be applied within families where sufficient family members are available for study to enable the laboratory to determine which individual markers are associated with the mutation-bearing chromosome. This is a serious restriction since in some families the critical members may not be available for study through geographical dispersal or, irrevocably, if the genetically determined disease is lethal.

There are also organizational and financial problems in performing complex laboratory tests on several members of an extended family. Further, such enquiries destroy the possibility of privacy for parents in relation to their decision on the taking of genetic risks.

Even when probes are available for the gene site itself (as with haemophilia or phenylketonuria), in practice gene markers may have to be used rather than tests for the mutation itself. This is because the *same disease* may result from many *different individual mutations* within the DNA complex that constitutes the gene. Unless the particular mutation for an individual family has been characterized in detail (which would be a very substantial task) it would not be possible to know with any precision which gene probe to apply. In the Lesch Nyhan syndrome, for example, a disorder of uric acid metabolism resulting in the subject being incapacitated by grossly abnormal movements with a strange proclivity to self-mutilation, eight cases have been characterized in detail and eight different gene mutations found.

These practical considerations are of major future importance since the approach to the eradication of genetically determined diseases will be different for those diseases whose population frequency is maintained by a high mutation rate (e.g. Duchenne muscular dystrophy) compared with those in which a relatively few ancestral mutation events have spread through a population (e.g. sickle cell anaemia and probably beta-thalassaemia). Thus, in the beta-thalassaemia example, where mutation rates are low, an approach to eradication of the disorder can in principle be based on screening large numbers of people to detect carriers. Such an approach has successfully led to a substantial decrease in the birth incidence of this disorder in some parts of the world. In Duchenne muscular dystrophy, where it is likely that one-third of all cases are new mutants born to non-carrier mothers, screening for carriers among those related to a known case, if such a scheme were introduced, could not reduce the disease incidence by more than two-thirds. The remainder could only be eradicated if reliable tests were available for mass screening of the fetus early in pregnancy.

Some of the disorders for which gene probes are available are shown in Table 2.1. This list is likely to grow very rapidly over the next few years.

Strategies for the prevention of congenital and hereditary disorders

Medical treatment usually begins with identifying the individual symptoms and signs of a particular disorder and finally making the diagnosis.

The usual approach to prevention of congenital and genetic disease starts with defining populations at high relative risk of having affected children. Different disorders can lend themselves to screening and preventive actions at different stages of a child's development, from the postnatal apparently normally formed but susceptible infant backwards through fetal life to considerations of the 'at risk' ovum and sperm.

Primary prevention

Primary prevention means the prevention of fetal abnormality by taking steps to protect the mother at risk, by preventing conception, or by counselling high-risk families who then choose to avoid further pregnancies. There are thus a number of approaches to primary prevention.

Where a disorder is known to result from a major environmental factor, avoidance of the relevant factor will prevent the disease. Rubella ('German measles') embryopathy and, in a somewhat different sense, rhesus immunization are examples of such congenital disorders which are open to primary prevention. If women enter the reproductive period already protected against rubella, either by having earlier suffered from the disease or being immunized against it, they will not contract the infection during pregnancy and will not therefore pass it on to their unborn child. The 15 per cent of women whose blood is rhesus negative (i.e. who possess a particular type of blood group), unlike those whose blood is rhesus positive, have a chance, if the father of the fetus is rhesus positive, of having infants affected by rhesus incompatibility in subsequent pregnancies as a result of 'antibodies' produced in the first pregnancy. Treatment of the mother (see p. 258) can almost eliminate

Table 2.1

Some disorders for which gene probes, or linked probes, have been reported. (The quality of available information is uneven, and not all of the probes are currently suitable for clinical use.)

Adenosine deaminase deficiency
Congenital adrenal hyperplasia (21-hydroxylase deficiency)
Adult polycystic kidney disease
Alport syndrome
Amyloidosis
Familial amyloidotic polyneuropathy
Antithrombin III deficiency
Alpha-1-antitrypsin deficiency
Apolipoprotein CII deficiency
Carbamyl phosphate synthetase I deficiency
Charcot−Marie−Tooth disease
Chorionic somatomammotropin deficiency
XL choroideremia
XL chronic granulomatous disease
Citrullinaemia
Cystic fibrosis
XL ectodermal dysplasia
Ehlers-Danlos syndrome
Factor X deficiency
Type I Gaucher disease
G6PD deficiency
Growth hormone deficiency type I
Haemophilia A
Haemophilia B
Hunter syndrome
Huntington's chorea
Familial hypercholesterolaemia
XL hypohidrotic ectodermal dysplasia
XL ichthyosis
Immunoglobulin K-chain deficiency
Lesch−Nyhan syndrome
Menkes kinky-hair disease
XL muscular dystrophies:
    Becker
    Duchenne
    Emery-Dreifuss
Myotonic dystrophy
Norrie's disease
OTC deficiency
Osteogenesis imperfecta type II
Phenylketonuria
XL retinitis pigmentosa
Sickle cell anaemia
α and β thalassaemia
von Willebrand disease
XL mental retardation

XL = X linked

the chance of her infants being affected by a disease which can kill or result in deafness, cerebral palsy, and mental handicap.

Many multifactorial disorders with a strong environmental component offer the possibility of manipulating the environment to prevent the expression of a disorder despite a susceptible genotype (inherent genetic constitution). Such an example of primary prevention is careful preconceptional blood glucose control among women with diabetes mellitus and the maintenance of such control throughout pregnancy. This is likely to reduce the higher than normal rate of malformation among infants born to mothers with diabetes. Similar benefit derives from treatment of mothers with phenylketonuria to control their blood phenylalanine (a derivative of dietary protein) levels during preconception and early gestation. These considerations clearly merge into areas of conventional health-care advice in pregnancy, such as the avoidance of cigarette smoking, excessive alcohol intake, and the taking of drugs which might damage the fetus. The suggestion, not yet completely proven, that preconceptional vitamin supplementation reduces the incidence of neural tube defects such as spina bifida would also come into the primary prevention category.

The approach to primary prevention is more complex for the majority of predominantly genetically determined disorders. Genetic counselling, informing parents at high risk of conceiving a genetically abnormal baby, is likely to lead to some such couples restricting their family size (Bobrow 1978).

In order to offer genetic counselling, 'at risk' couples must be identified. Generally, for the common recessive diseases like cystic fibrosis or phenylketonuria, this only happens *after* the birth of an affected child. Even were there to be 100 per cent efficiency in case detection and subsequent avoidance of recurrence within these families suffering from recessively inherited disorders, the effect on the incidence of such disorders in our society as a whole would be limited. The only chance of such primary prevention for the population as a whole would be a systematic screening to detect carriers of abnormal genes before they have affected offspring, plus counselling against pregnancy. Such an undertaking would only be justified for fairly common yet serious conditions for which accurate carrier tests were available. Screening for rhesus negative women was an early example of this practice. Population screening for thalassaemias in Sardinia, Italy, and Greece has resulted in a substantial number of couples being identified and informed of their carrier status. Most of these have proceeded to screening of their conceptus for homozygous disease (the type of the disease which will affect the child seriously) with termination of pregnancy if this is revealed. Population screening for other diseases is also possible; for example, for sickle cell disease in blacks and for Tay Sachs disease among Ashkenazi Jews.

It remains to be seen to what extent different societies will find such an approach to the eradication of genetically determined disease acceptable. We shall return to this subject at the end of the Chapter.

Secondary prevention

This term refers to the prevention of the live birth of an affected fetus by prenatal diagnosis and the termination of pregnancy.

Prenatal diagnosis Techniques allowing diagnosis of some fetal abnormalities (whether of genetic or environmental origin) have evolved greatly during the past decade and have become a routine part of obstetric care. The fetus may be examined directly by ultrasound, a non-invasive method of visualizing the fetus using ultrasound waves, or, if indicated, by fetoscopy (the fetoscope is an optical tube passed into the mother's uterus which allows direct visualization of the fetus). Fetal tissue may be removed by amniocentesis (removal of a sample of amniotic fluid from the mother's uterus), by venesection (removal of blood from a vein), or by direct biopsy (removal of a piece of tissue). Amniocentesis is thought to carry a risk of between 0.5 and 1 per cent of fetal death, and fetoscopic procedures slightly higher than this. There are no documented hazards of obstetric ultrasound but large-scale controlled trials testing the safety of ultrasound have not been conducted.

The fetus may also be examined indirectly, for example by screening maternal serum for alpha-fetoprotein (AFP), a type of protein found in raised amounts in maternal blood in the presence of neural tube defects such as spina bifida and abdominal wall defects (Wald, Cuckle, Brock, Peto, Polani, and Woodford 1977; Clarke, Gordan, Kitan, Chard, and Letchworth 1977).

The diagnosis of abnormality may occasionally lead to treatment. For example, in the case of rhesus disease, transfusion of blood through the mother's abdominal wall directly into the peritonal cavity of the fetus, or plasmapheresis of the mother (a process of removing antibodies from the mother's circulation), may allow the pregnancy to proceed long enough for the fetus to reach a level of maturity to allow delivery and survival. More often, however, the abnormalities detected are not open to treatment and the parents are faced with the choice of allowing the malformed pregnancy to continue or be terminated.

When dealing with conditions for which no treatment is available, the pregnant woman and her husband, before embarking on prenatal diagnostic tests, need to receive expert counselling on the implications and the decisions they may have to face arising from the tests. Although many pregnant women submit themselves to prenatal diagnosis in the expectation and hope that it will prove normality, they may do so without having made a final decision on what action they will take should an abnormality be discovered. In practice, however, it is a rarity for a pregnancy tested for, and shown to have, a major abnormality such as Down's syndrome not to be terminated.

Mid-trimester diagnosis and termination of pregnancy Mid-trimester diagnosis and termination of pregnancy by amniocentesis, usually at 16–18 weeks gestation or later, is an unsatisfactory solution to the problem of congenital abnormality. However, the continually increasing referral rates for amniocentesis suggest a wide public acceptance of this approach in the absence of more attractive alternatives. Since the procedure involves some risks, it can only be applied to defined high-risk populations. The common criteria of eligibility include a high maternal serum AFP level (which identifies a risk of fetal abnormality of between 5 and 10 per cent), a family history of a diagnosable disorder, and advanced maternal age (which confers an increased risk of Down's syndrome and most other chromosomal trisomies—the presence in each body cell of an extra chromosome, an abnormality which is usually associated with a variety of serious disorders).

Serum AFP screening has led to a noticeable decrease in the frequency of neural tube defect births (Wald and Cuckle 1984). The magnitude of the decrease is difficult to calculate, however, because it is superimposed on a large and unexplained downward trend in the incidence of neural tube defects unrelated to this procedure. The effect of screening for Down's syndrome is more difficult to determine as routine population data are not collected. A policy of screening pregnant women over the age of 35 years, if taken up by half of those eligible, would be expected to reduce the incidence of the disorder by about 15 per cent in the population as a whole. Although older women are at a higher risk, most Down's syndrome babies are in fact the products of the low risk but much more numerous pregnancies of younger women.

Early prenatal diagnosis and the termination of pregnancy   Prenatal diagnosis at 16–18 weeks of gestation has obvious medical, social, and psychological disadvantages. Once a pregnancy is physically evident and particularly once fetal movements are perceived, the parents, perhaps specially the mother, may be unable easily to countenance the death of the fetus. Termination of the pregnancy much earlier in gestation is likely to be generally more acceptable.

The technique of chorion villus sampling (CVS) enables a wide range of investigations to be performed between eight and ten weeks of gestation. The technique involves passing a catheter through the cervix of the uterus to the placental bed under ultrasonic guidance, following which about 20 mg of chorionic tissue (part of the placenta or afterbirth) is aspirated. The material can then be used for a variety of analyses either by direct processing or by growing the fetal cells in tissue culture prior to analysis. This is possible because the cytotrophoblast (the early placenta) is an actively proliferating tissue the dividing cells of which are suitable for chromosome analysis. The chorionic biopsy samples can also be processed directly for DNA analysis. Additionally, various enzyme assays can be performed either on the tissue sample itself or on the cells cultured from it. The DNA analysis and enzyme assays will require to be investigated disease by disease since there is no single test which will measure the normality of the conceptus. This restriction applies equally to mid-trimester and postnatal diagnostic techniques.

Current estimates suggest that up to 3 per cent of pregnancies miscarry after CVS. This is likely to be a maximal figure as the technique is still relatively new. Nothing is yet known on the long-term side-effects of CVS. These will only become apparent in postnatal life with the careful follow-up of babies whose earlier gestation had been subject to this technique. It seems likely that

CVS will largely replace amniocentesis in the coming years. This may lead to some increase in public acceptance of prenatal diagnosis. There will however be major organizational problems in arranging for large numbers of pregnancies to be referred to specialist centres before the tenth week of gestation.

With the extension of the repertoire of prenatal diagnosis *couples at risk of genetically determined disorders* may undertake further pregnancies with the clear understanding that an abnormal pregnancy (abnormal fetus) may be terminated. There will be, among their normal fetuses, 'carrier' offspring who will be clinically well. This could, under some circumstances, lead to a very slow net increase in the frequencies of abnormal genes in our society. From the physician's point of view it seems more appropriate to concentrate on the immediate problems of the family rather than on the longer term problems of society. In practice, it is impossible for the clinician to weigh the possibility of increasing the frequency of genetically determined disease in several hundred years' time against the immediate needs of his patients.

Tertiary prevention

Tertiary prevention might serve as a useful term to include postnatal environmental manipulation with a view to the avoidance of the effects of genetically determined disease. Dietary regulation in the treatment of phenylketonuria might come under this heading: without dietary regulation the baby will suffer progressive and severe dementia. With a phenylalanine-regulated synthetic diet the same baby can be expected to grow up to be a mentally normal child and adult. Other disorders, apart from such clearly defined inborn errors of metabolism, may come into this category. For example, if it is shown that diabetes mellitus results from an identifiable environmental factor afflicting the genetically susceptible individual, this would offer the chance of factor avoidance or immunization in the prevention of the disease.

Postnatal screening

Screening is commonly conducted in the postnatal period to identify phenylketonuria and congenital hypothyroidism (cretinism). Both of these conditions can be diagnosed from small blood samples taken in the first week or two after birth; they are both relatively common (in the order of one case every 5000 to 10 000 births) and both are amenable to therapeutic manoeuvres—in the case of phenylketonuria a synthetic diet low in phenylalanine and in the case of hypothyroidism supplements of the missing hormone thyroxine.

It is technically possible to identify cystic fibrosis and Duchenne muscular dystrophy immediately after birth. Although there is evidence that early diagnosis of cystic fibrosis may result in improved management and subsequent prognosis (which is not the case with muscular dystrophy), neither of these conditions is 'curable'. Early diagnosis might be considered here to be largely concerned with alerting the couple that they are at high risk of future pregnancies being affected. It has been estimated that around 10 per cent of pregnancies affected by Duchenne muscular dystrophy might be avoided in this way.

In vitro fertilization

There is no technical reason why the principle of early prenatal diagnosis should not be capable of further development. Embryos developed *in vitro* from the sperm and ova of high-risk couples can be studied. A few cells could be taken for testing at an early stage in embryogenesis, before the cells are committed to particular developmental pathways. The feasibility and safety of this manoeuvre is illustrated by the fact that monozygotic (identical) twins represent early embryonic splitting, each component of the split being compatible with normal development into the full individual. Embryonic cells removed could be studied, either directly or after culture, for their chromosomal and genetic make-up and only 'normal' embryos implanted into the mother. Thus at the cost of some considerable technical interference with conception and early pregnancy, such *in vitro* testing could, in principle, eliminate the need for CVS or mid-trimester prenatal diagnosis.

Whether this approach would meet with wide public acceptability depends on the efficiency and reliability of the techniques and the extent to which the procedure can be improved so as to minimize intrusion into the private lives of the couples concerned.

Considerations for society

Congenital and genetically determined disorders are becoming increasingly prominent causes of childhood morbidity and mortality in industrialized societies, as malnutrition and infectious diseases are controlled. Regrettably we still understand little of their primary aetiology, and the nature of the defects is such that they do not readily lend themselves to treatment. While primary prevention is applicable to a small proportion of the problems, the only practical approach available in many situations depends on secondary prevention.

Secondary prevention, the prevention of live birth of an affected conceptus, poses complex ethical choices for society and for the individuals concerned. There are two levels at which society must judge these developments, the physical and the psycho–social–ethical. On the purely physical side we must be certain that new procedures are not introduced until their safety and efficacy have been carefully and objectively assessed. At a time when the escalating costs of health care are giving rise to concern, some form of cost-benefit analysis also has to be made. If resources do not allow all forms of available health care to be delivered to all sectors of society, the decisions about which restrictions to impose must be social and political decisions rather than primarily medical ones. Consider, for example, the impact of the following: the estimated cost of caring for a severely disabled person (with Down's syndrome, for example) is currently about £10 000 per annum or £300 000 over the lifetime of the individual. Although such accounting is fraught with difficulties and is dehumanizing, it seems likely that any prevention of congenital disability which can be achieved will be justifiable in economic terms. We must then consider in turn how that cost-saving exercise may affect society's judgement in humanitarian and ethical terms.

The procedures discussed in this chapter will have some long-term effects on the frequencies of abnormal genes in the population, but the effects are unlikely to be dramatic. Couples informed that they are at a high genetic risk tend to have fewer children. Couples caring for a disabled child may be discouraged from further pregnancies. Couples who terminate an abnormal pregnancy may replace it fairly rapidly. For recessive diseases, there is a two-out-of-three chance that such normal children as they have will be carriers of the abnormal gene. These practices could therefore lead to a gradual rise in abnormal gene frequencies. The time-scale for noticeable change will be in the order of hundreds or even thousands of years. Nevertheless it would seem reasonable to hold a watching brief on the outcome of some of the preventive procedures until more factual information becomes available. Of much more immediate and significant importance is the change in gene frequency which will come about with the longer survival into their reproductive years of affected individuals, such as those with haemophilia and cystic fibrosis.

On the ethical side a variety of obvious concerns have been expressed. The most straightforward of these relates to the termination of abnormal pregnancies. Some people find any termination of pregnancy unacceptable. A majority of our society (in the Western industrial world at least) regard termination as reasonable in the face of severe untreatable abnormality. However, individuals and society at large find infanticide unacceptable; in pregnancy there must therefore be a point between 18 weeks and birth when for most people the boundary of acceptability is crossed. Intuitively, an increasing value is placed on a fetus as it grows more closely to resemble a new-born baby. Furthermore, advances in intensive perinatal care have conferred a 90 per cent chance of survival on babies live-born who are normally formed at 28 weeks gestation; and a 50 per cent chance of survival for the infant born after a gestation as short as 25–26 weeks. As a result it might be judged that the 'value' attributed to the life of the fetus after 20 weeks gestation will progressively increase with the progressive success of postnatal intensive care.

Conversely, the technical advances facilitating termination, the increased precision of prenatal diagnosis, and the general availability of such techniques as obstetric ultrasound have reduced the perceived value of the life of the fetus below (say) 18 weeks gestation.

First trimester fetal diagnosis has generally been welcomed, giving rise to a shift in the focus of our dilemma further backwards in gestation towards the issue of the selection of early embryos and *in vitro* fertilization. It is perhaps too soon to be formulating a consensus view of society on these matters. However, the fact that the technology is advancing very rapidly might indicate that a consensus view is urgently required.

Technical advances are relatively easy to describe and appreciate. The abstract components of the associated dilemmas and the value that individuals and society put on human life are weighty matters for discussion even among the wisest of physicians, philosophers, and theologians. Undoubtedly, we have an increasing capacity for technical intervention in human reproduction, spanning from before conception through to childbirth. It behoves us to consider the effects these developments may have on parenthood itself (with its demands for selfless devotion to the baby and dependent infant), on family life, and on other aspects of human social behaviour. We know little about the effects of genetic counselling and prenatal diagnosis on subsequent marital stability, for example, yet we have intruded into an area of human behaviour which is intensely private. It seems unlikely that medical interference in this area of fundamental human behaviour will be without some effects.

Nevertheless there is every sign that the attempts to tackle the problem of congenital and hereditary disease, along the lines discussed in this chapter, enjoy reasonably widespread support in this country. It remains to be seen whether the technologically developed world's opinion develops and remains uniform on these issues. While the media can disseminate information as never before, and while the routine provision of new diagnostic and therapeutic techniques tends to diffuse the ethical dilemmas that surround them, we should nevertheless take time to recognize the velocity with which human reproductive technology is advancing. We might question who, if anyone, might be wise enough to hold this advance in check.

As a final thought towards achieving the best balance in this infinitely complex equation, we should perhaps remember that clinical advances are being made in the treatment of children born alive with genetically determined diseases. There is a gene probe for phenylketonuria: this would allow CVS and termination of pregnancy; however, such children, with a synthetic balanced diet, grow to be normal adults. There is a gene probe for cystic fibrosis: a few years ago, such children had a life expectancy little beyond ten years; even now such children's life expectancy appears to be nearer 20 years and in some centres nearer 30. There is every likelihood that further advances in therapy will in time become available. It is therefore important to ensure that the right balance is maintained between the continuing exploration of improvements in therapy and the deceptive administrative simplicity of secondary prevention.

References

Bobrow, M. (1978). Genetic counselling: a tool for the prevention of some abnormal pregnancies. *Journal of Clinical Pathology* **29** (suppl. 10), pp. 145-9.

Clarke, P. C., Gordon, Y. D., Kitan, M. J., Chard, T., and Letchworth, A. T. (1977). Screening for neural tube defects by maternal plasma alpha feto-protein determinations. *British Journal of Obstetrics and Gynaecology* **84**, pp. 568-73.

Emery, A. E. H. and Rimoin, D. L. (1983). Nature and incidence of genetic disease. In *Principles and practice of medical genetics*, pp. 1-3. Churchill Livingstone, Edinburgh.

Kaback, M. M. (1984). . In *The utility of prenatal diagnosis* (eds. C. H. Rodeck and K. H. Nicolaides), pp. 1-12. Royal College of Obstetricians and Gynaecologists.

Roberts, D. F., Shavez, J., and Court, S. D. M. (1970). Genetic component in childhood mortality. *Archives of Disease in Childhood* **45**, pp. 33-8.

Wald, N. J. and Cuckle, H. (1984). Open neural tube defects. In *Antenatal and neonatal screening*, pp. 25-73. Oxford University Press. Oxford.

Wald, N. J., Cuckle, H., Brock, D. J. H., Peto, R., Polani, P. E., and Woodford, F. T. (1977). UK collaborative study on maternal serum alpha-protein measurement in antenatal screening for anencephaly and spina bifida in early pregnancy. *Lancet* **1**, pp. 1323-32.

3

The care of new-born babies—some developments and dilemmas

RICHARD W. I. COOKE and PAMELA A. DAVIES

Historical aspects

Founding members of the British Paediatric Association (BPA) were little involved with the care of babies in 1928. These doctors (in reality physicians who were engaged predominantly in adult medicine but in addition had a special interest in diseases of children) were few in number, and their influence did not extend to the new-born nursery. This was the province of devoted and authoritarian nursing staff, who turned to obstetricians for help if necessary. In 1931, the country's first special nursery for premature infants was opened in the grounds of the Sorrento Maternity Hospital, Birmingham. It owed its existence to the initiative and drive of a pioneering public health doctor, Mary Crosse, who was to gain renown for her work and teaching there. The BPA's first public pronouncement on the new-born baby was its report *Neonatal Mortality*, submitted to an extraordinary general meeting in 1942. This clearly identified areas of concern, and called for more teaching and for properly equipped, and efficiently staffed, neonatal units in each maternity hospital and in most of the larger children's hospitals. Acknowledging that the problems of neonatal mortality (deaths occurring in the first 27 days of life) concerned general practitioners, public health workers, and general physicians as well as obstetricians and paediatricians, it urged the latter to accept the onus of leadership in tackling the problem. The report was to be the forerunner of many similar, if lengthier, documents stemming from working parties over the next 40 years requesting the same improvements.

Although a few children's doctors had gained a tenuous foothold in new-born nurseries in some parts of the country during the Second World War, the advent of the National Health Service in

1948 gave greater impetus to the move into the maternity departments. Relations with obstetricians were often uneasy in the early days, but a paediatric presence became an accepted fact over the next ten years. Nursing staff continued to play an important role, for paediatricians and young doctors in training had to divide their time between the new-born baby and the older child. In retrospect this first decade was not an auspicious one. The newly available antimicrobial drugs and other treatments were prescribed for the first time often over-lavishly in attempts to lower mortality, and some salutory lessons in developmental physiology and pharmacology were learned the hard way. But the experimental work of physiologists and clinical scientists such as Barcroft, Cross, Dawes, Huggett, McCance, and Widdowson helped clinicians towards a more rational basis for their work. The growing interest in new-born infants was further fostered by the formation of the Neonatal Society in 1959, which provided a forum where they could meet.

The last 20 of the BPA's first 60 years have seen the greatest changes as technology has been harnessed to neonatal care. The sick new-born infant is now warmed, fed, ventilated, and monitored by a plethora of electronically controlled equipment (Plates XIV, XV, and XVI). The administration of this care has become more dependent on doctors, and exclusively neonatal posts have become available as part of junior doctors' training in paediatrics. Consultant paediatricians too may practise neonatology only, though numbers doing so are still small. Successful application of the new care would never have been achieved without a parallel expansion of nurse training. As survival has increased, so parental expectations have grown, and perceptions of parents' needs and feelings by medical and nursing staff can be said to be more acute than at any time previously.

Certain hospitals have been designated as regional centres for neonatal intensive care, and mothers are transferred to these hospitals for delivery if problems such as extreme prematurity of the infant are anticipated. Alternatively, though less preferable, infants may be transported to the centres after birth with intensive support on the journey by a trained team. This is a far cry from the days when babies arrived at the newly built Sorrento unit 'fetched by a nurse in a taxi with a basket fitted up with hot water bottles'.

Falling mortality rates

The perinatal and neonatal mortality rates[1] have fallen steadily in almost every developed country since the earlier part of this century. Death around the time of birth is mainly related to low birth-weight, birth asphyxia, and lethal congenital abnormalities. Although these problems would appear amenable in many cases to medical intervention, the contribution of improvements in perinatal care to the reduction in mortality is far from clear. For instance, it has been estimated that as much as one-third of the reduction in perinatal mortality in recent years may be attributed to fertility control.

Low birth-weight (less than 2.5 kg) is the major contributor to perinatal and neonatal mortality. The proportion of such infants born in England and Wales during the past 30 years has not altered significantly, remaining at 6–7 per cent. Low-birth-weight-specific neonatal mortality figures for England and Wales have been available since 1953, grouped as shown in Fig. 3.1, and from 1963 it has been possible to separate the birth-weights of those 1.5 kg and under into those above and below 1 kg. Figure 3.1 shows, however, that in all low-birth-weight groupings there has been an accelerated decline in mortality since about 1975. Although there may be some demographic changes to explain this there seems every reason to suppose that neonatal intensive care has played the major part in this increased survival.

Some very low-birth-weight deaths now occur beyond the first 27 days while the infants are still in hospital, and the post-neonatal mortality rate (one month to one year) compared with the neonatal mortality rate has not declined to anything like the same degree. Transfer to the post-neonatal period for infants who previously would have died in the neonatal period cannot account, however, for the marked decreases in neonatal mortality rates.

Although the low-birth-weight rate for the country as a whole has remained unchanged, significant improvements in the low-birth-weight rate have been made locally in a number of cases by social and medical interventions. In a trial in Edinburgh, decentralization and reorganization of antenatal care by general practitioners in co-operation with obstetricians improved uptake of

[1] Perinatal mortality rate: deaths occurring between 28 weeks of gestation and less than seven completed days from birth per 1000 total births. Neonatal mortality rate: deaths occurring during the first 27 days of life per 1000 live births.

Congenital malformations

Relative importance and ethical problems

While infants with congenital malformations contribute about 25 per cent of deaths at or around the time of birth, a substantial number survive into childhood and beyond. The reduction in mortality from low birth-weight, with improvements in neonatal intensive care, makes malformation increasingly important as a cause of death and disability. Whilst the actual cause of most malformations remains unknown, it is important to realize that malformed infants at birth represent only the 'tip of the iceberg' of congenital abnormality in that the vast majority of abnormal conceptions are lost before maturity. This quality control of nature results in nearly half of all conceptions being lost before term. The mechanism of this process of 'teratothanasia' is unknown, but its recognition can be used to justify the process of antenatal diagnosis and abortion of identified abnormal fetuses on the grounds that such procedures simply carry on where nature failed to identify malformation.

The use of ultrasound scanning in particular has allowed the identification of a wide range of malformations at 16–20 weeks of pregnancy. This technique involves very short 'sound' waves whose pattern and 'echo' on impinging on deep body organs can reveal their size and structure. Spinal, cardiac, renal, and gastro-intestinal malformations are easily diagnosed by the skilled ultrasonographer; so are more minor abnormalities such as limb deformities and cleft lip and palate, which may be compatible with a normal life-style after surgical correction. To date it has not proved economical in most centres to offer detailed ultrasound screening of every fetus whose mother would wish it, but, even if this were feasible, considerable ethical problems would arise. What degree of abnormality should justify termination of pregnancy? Many malformations even of the heart or gut are relatively easily treated surgically after birth. With many parents electing to bear only one or two children, the pressure to have only normal children is greater and the tolerance of abnormality less. How small an abnormality can justify pregnancy termination, and who should make this decision?

The psychological effects of elective (as opposed to spontaneous) pregnancy termination should not be underestimated. A recent study relating to antenatal diagnosis of spina bifida showed a much higher incidence of depression in mothers after abortion of an abnormal fetus than was seen in a group of mothers experiencing pregnancy termination for social reasons.

Can malformations be prevented rather than simply terminated? At least 70 per cent of congenital malformations are of unknown cause, usually being described as 'multifactorial' or 'polygenic' in origin. These terms imply genetic abnormality involving a number of genes of a type where environmental influences as well as potential genetic abnormality are likely to combine to cause an overt congenital defect. Empirical observations may lead to the development of theories of causation; for example, in a disease such as spina bifida, where circumstantial evidence suggests that dietary deficiencies may interact with a genetic predisposition. Unfortunately, in this instance, poorly designed studies involving small numbers of patients have resulted in inconclusive results, and the role of folate deficiency suspected as a possible cause of spina bifida remains undetermined (folate is an essential ingredient of diet and must be present in adequate amounts).

A small number of malformations (less than 5 per cent) are related to viral infections during pregnancy. Rubella infection (German measles) in pregnancy is essentially preventable by immunization, but uptake by schoolgirls is too low to be completely effective. Immunization of both sexes in early childhood so that widespread immunity lowers the incidence of the disease in the community, as practised in the USA, may be more effective if the uptake of immunization is higher at this time. Unfortunately other important viral infections such as that by the cytomegalovirus are not yet preventable by immunization. Cytomegalovirus infection is an infection which may occur in the mother during pregnancy with little or no disturbance but may be transmitted by her to the fetus resulting, in a few cases only, in jaundice and haemorrhage in the infant at birth and in residual damage to the brain and eyes if the infant lives. Fortunately most fetuses escape such impairment.

The absence of credible explanations for most congenital malformations has led to the spawning of many theories which verge on the incredible. Certain paramedical groups have widely publicized certain unproved and scientifically dubious theories, mostly based on the presence or absence of various trace metals in body fluids. Perhaps only a fuller understanding of the randomness of some of the earlier events in the development of the human fetus will put these speculations into perspective.

Surgical treatment

Advances in anaesthetic and surgical techniques and improvements in post-operative care have increased the scope of neonatal surgery and have allowed infants with previously lethal malformations to survive. Surgeons, like neonatalogists, have tackled increasingly more difficult problems in the knowledge that the full implications of their endeavours could not be evident for many years. Some malformations may be corrected and others only modified. The resulting quality of life may vary considerably. As parents have become more aware of the likely outcome, many have wished to become involved in the clinical decision-making, rather than leaving this to the medical profession alone. Some of the dilemmas of recent years in judging the pros and cons of different neonatal surgical procedures are exemplified in the changing attitudes to the treatment of spina bifida.

Spina bifida and hydrocephalus　　Most babies born with spina bifida used to die untreated in early infancy either from infection or from progressive hydrocephalus. Thirty years ago the Spitz–Holter valve was developed which allowed this excess of cerebrospinal fluid or 'water on the brain' to be shunted away to a blood vessel or to the peritoneal cavity where it could be absorbed. Shortly after the introduction of this device a policy of immediate closure of the back lesion and shunt insertion later, as needed, was started in some centres in this country. By 1971 it was clear that while mortality was progressively decreasing the large majority of the survivors had major physical defects and were often mentally retarded. The outlook was worst for those babies in whom hydrocephalus and kyphosis (a deformity of the spine) were already apparent at birth, in addition to the extensive paralysis.

　　A more selective approach to surgery was introduced in the early 1970s as these results became known. Infants born with the most extensive lesions were not operated upon unless their parents expressly wished it. It was assumed that death would occur early, and if the babies were nursed in hospital it usually did. However, when parents undertook care at home, as they were encouraged and supported in so doing in some centres, a proportion of the babies survived. In Newcastle-upon-Tyne, for instance, shunt surgery was undertaken as needed later and cosmetic surgery for the back lesion later still. At school entry, these survivors were wheelchair bound and incontinent, but not mentally retarded, perhaps because they were not hydrocephalic at birth. Most were no more disabled than others who had been operated on immediately. These results showed that survival and prevention of later disability did not depend on immediate operation, and that time was available for comprehensive discussion and support for parents who did not need to be faced with an irreversible life-or-death decision at birth.

In the early years in which immediate surgery was performed for spina bifida the problems of treatment were not confined to the neonatal period. There were repeated hospital admissions for shunt revisions; recurrent infections occurred; orthopaedic procedures were often required; and some form of urinary diversion (surgical operation on the urinary system) was often practised in an effort to improve urinary continence. Later, major social problems arose as these children grew up. Today the picture is less gloomy, with an 85 per cent survival rate for surgery; the intelligence for many comes within the normal range and urinary continence with the aid of intermittent catheterization can usually be achieved. New devices may allow more to walk. The ability of families to meet the challenge of a disabled child, however, can vary enormously and many feel that the help provided is wholly inadequate and the burden which they and their handicapped child carry ill-appreciated. Effective support is essential not just in the early years but throughout adolescence and adult life as well.

Congenital heart disease   Heart defects comprise one of the largest groups of congenital malformations. The formerly greatly restricted and shortened lives of some children with severe congenital heart disease have been transformed by cardiac surgery in recent years to lives of normal or near normal activity and span. This era began just over 50 years ago when the first patent *ductus arteriosus* was ligated. This channel between the two main arteries of the heart occasionally remains open, as in fetal life, when it serves to shunt blood away from the fluid-filled lungs. Normally it should close soon after birth so that the blood may be routed through the expanding lungs which take over the essential task of supplying the blood with oxygen. In the past 20 years the techniques of cardiopulmonary bypass (oxygenating the blood by an extracorporeal machine while the heart, empty of blood, is operated on) and deep hypothermia (profound but controlled cooling of the patient) have allowed surgeons much greater scope with access to the inside of the heart. The advent of two-dimensional ultrasound, together with Doppler velocimetry (a means of estimating the flow of blood), have augmented angiography (radiological outlining of blood vessels) as diagnostic tools of increasing precision. These new methods have been of first importance to the new-born infant for, although only a small proportion of heart surgery is conducted in the neonatal period, it is often needed urgently.

Although a diagnosis of heart disease can be made before birth, the much more specific and precise techniques for diagnosis after birth and the wider availability of these postnatal services mean that an infant who may benefit from prompt surgery has to be identified in this way. As the greatest risk to survival in congenital heart disease extends throughout the first year, it is difficult or impossible to separate the neonatal period from the ensuing 11 months in discussing outcome. It is not surprising that few population studies are available, for cardiac surgery is practised in relatively few centres, which may receive their patients from a wide area. The outcome of 599 infants surviving three or more weeks after operation in the first year of life and studied at the Institute of Child Health in London over the 25 years up to 1976 has been presented in the form of actuarial survival curves for each operation for a given condition. This method of analysis allows the likelihood of late survival to be calculated during the period over which operations are being carried out. Four operative risk categories were established, high survival rate or low survival rate, early only or late survival. The results showed the superiority of one-stage over two-stage repair for transposition of the great arteries (a severe but relatively common disorder in which the aorta arises from the right ventricle and the pulmonary artery from the left, instead of vice versa) and for ventricular septal defect (a hole in the septum between the two ventricles of the heart) with early and late survival exceeding 90 per cent. The authors point out that these operations on new-born infants have in no case been without some long-term complications or mortality. Some operations have had to be repeated later—for example coarctation (narrowing) of the aorta in which recoarctation occurred. The results of surgery, however, are infinitely superior to medical treatment in a number of lesions in which death would have occurred before the end of the first year of life (Macartney, Taylor, Graham, de Leval, and Stark 1980).

Survival is likely to increase further in the next 25 years, with the use of newer supporting medical treatments such as pre-operative prostaglandin E infusions to augment pulmonary blood flow where complex operations on conditions such as pulmonary atresia (blockage of blood flow to the lungs due to an imperforate pulmonary artery) with intact septum are being carried out. Improvement of surgical techniques will include attempts to preserve the entire cardiac conduction system (the 'electrical' system which controls co-ordination of the pumping action of the heart) during operations to lessen the likelihood of the later development of cardiac arrhythmias (disturbances of pumping rhythm) with their inherent danger of sudden death. It is unfortunate that for some babies the ability to correct or at least palliate their heart lesion has been accompanied by cerebrovascular accidents ('strokes') either during surgery or due to polycythaemia. This thickening of the blood due to an increased number of red cells is a compensatory mechanism for its poor oxygenation in certain types of serious congenital heart disease, and unfortunately increases the risk of clotting or thrombosis. The prevalence of such problems is small, however.

Although ethical problems do not occur to the same extent in the treatment of congenital heart disease as in the treatment of spina bifida, controversy sometimes arises over the treatment of children with Down's syndrome of whom 40 per cent have heart defects. One-third of these defects are partial or complete atrioventricular canals (inadequate separation of the pumping chambers of the heart so that they leak into each other). Children with complete defect will die by five years with medical treatment alone and will fail to thrive, becoming progressively more cyanosed (blue) and breathless before death. Compassion dictates that they should be offered surgery in the same way as a normal child. Seventy-five per cent may be expected to survive surgery and their life span is then likely to be that of Down's syndrome in general (20–40 years or more). The BPA considers that in the case of a malformed infant its members will first attend to the needs of the infant but will at the same time have a concern for the family as a whole. There must be few who would not consider surgery for Down's syndrome babies with congenital gastro-intestinal lesions such as atresia or blind-ending of the oesophagus (gullet) or duodenum (part of the gut just below the stomach), unless other conditions such as extremely low birth-weight are also present.

Low birth-weight

Factors influencing survival

The failure of the low-birth-weight rate to fall in the past 30 years or so is disappointing. Over the period in which information has been available there has been no substantial change in the distribution of births within the weight groupings shown in Fig. 3.1. In 1980, for example, nearly 7 per cent of all live births were less than 2.5 kg in weight, and 0.2 per cent weighed less than 1.0 kg. There are regional variations. During 1978–1980 the lowest low-birth-weight rate in one regional health authority (South-West Thames region of London) was 6.1 per cent and the highest 8.0 per cent (North-West region), with fluctuations above and below these figures for individual districts within each region. While low-birth-weight rates show little change it is not possible to say whether the unchanging rate conceals within it any shift in the distribution of babies who are of low birth-weight because of pre-term birth or small because they have grown too slowly in the uterus. There are also national variations. Sweden, Norway, and New Zealand have low-birth-weight rates below 5 per cent, while the USA, Poland, the USSR, Hungary, and Cuba have rates above 7 per cent. Many less developed countries have significantly higher rates associated with increased rates of intra-uterine growth retardation. If a mother's country of origin is taken as a pointer to her ethnic origin, an analysis of low-birth-weight rates among infants born in England and Wales in 1980 showed that the highest rate (12.4 per cent) related to mothers born in the African Commonwealth, and the lowest (3.9 per cent) to those born in Australia, Canada, and New Zealand. Other high low-birth-weight rates were seen for infants born to mothers from India and Bangladesh, Pakistan, and the West Indies, the figures being 11.9, 10.5, and 9.0 per cent, respectively.

Low birth-weight is often divided into specific groups: less than 1.5, 1.5–1.999, and 2.0–2.499 kg. Infants are less commonly found in these groups when their fathers belong to the Registrar General's higher Social Classes—I, II, and III—and more commonly found when their fathers are in the lower social classes—IV and V. The highest rates are found in those recorded as illegitimate. Approximately ten-times as many multiple births as single births are of low birth-weight, but the perinatal mortality of low-birth-weight single births is higher than that of low-birth-weight multiple births. Although quadruplets and higher multiple births have increased somewhat since fertility drugs have been available, multiple births per 1000 total maternities have declined since the 1950s. More low-birth-weight babies are born on Saturdays and Sundays than on weekdays, and the perinatal mortality is also higher at weekends. Low-birth-weight males, though on average heavier than low-birth-weight females, have a higher mortality for any given gestational age (Macfarlane and Mugford 1984).

Present scope of care

The improvement in the survival of low-birth-weight infants in recent years may be attributed to a better understanding of their basic physiology, of the disease processes from which they suffer, and new technologies for diagnosis and treatment. Respiratory distress, mostly due to hyaline membrane disease (HMD) (obstruction of the small airways of the pre-term infant's lungs due to narrowing by a lining membrane: also associated with other disturbances of lung function), is both the commonest life-threatening disorder in pre-term babies and the condition in which the greatest progress in prevention and management in neonatology has been made in the past 25 years. Early ideas on the pathophysiology of HMD concentrated on inadequate blood flow through the lungs as a cause. Later, pathologists noted the low surface tension and tendency to foam possessed by fluid from normal lungs and the absence of these properties in fluid from lungs of infants dying from HMD. Further work then established the origin, function, and nature of these surface active·agents ('surfactants'). (Lack of surfactant results in some of the air cells of the lung collapsing and others being over-inflated with diminished lung function as a consequence.) Treatment with a synthetic surfactant in pre-term infants with HMD was initially tried over 20 years ago, but without success. The method of administration probably rendered the surfactant inactive. Further work in Cambridge, England in the 1970s resulted in the production and clinical trial of a more effective artificial surfactant mixture. Other centres in North America, Japan, and Scandinavia have also claimed success with a variety of surfactants extracted from animal lungs or from human amniotic fluid. None the less, surfactant trials have only reduced rather than replaced the need for other therapies.

The mainstay of management of HMD, apart from general supportive measures, is mechanical ventilation (MV). Early attempts at MV were relatively unsuccessful, partly because of the reluctance to ventilate infants before they were terminally ill and partly because the techniques used were inappropriate. Infants surviving the initial illness often became chronically ventilator dependent because of lung fibrosis and died later. Recognition that the degree of lung fibrosis was related to the ventilator inflation pressure used led to new approaches to ventilation pressures and timing which resulted in improvement both in the number of survivors and in their quality of life.

The value of a low constant positive pressure applied to the sick infant's airway during or instead of MV as a means of preventing negative pressure developing in the thorax during inspiration was shown in the early 1970s, and infant ventilators were redesigned to allow this to be done. Further modifications in ventilator therapy by using different rates of ventilation and muscle relaxants (to abolish the infant's own respiratory efforts which may 'fight' with the ventilator in that they are not synchronous with it) have been introduced to reduce the complication of lung rupture frequently seen with MV. Success in the treatment of larger pre-term infants has led to treatment being offered to ever smaller babies, and it is possible to apply MV to infants as small as 500 g. However, such attempts are inevitably associated with a higher mortality and an increased rate of both acute and long-term complications.

Although MV represents the major therapeutic intervention in the sick pre-term infant, its success or otherwise is extremely dependent on the ability to control the infant's whole environment by monitoring vital functions and providing a stable thermal environment and total nutritional requirements for periods of several weeks or even months. The development by the medical equipment industry of servo-controlled incubators (a probe attached to the baby regulates the heating of the incubator to maintain the baby's temperature at a predetermined level) and radiant warmers, electronic monitoring of heart rate, blood pressure, temperature, and respiration, and accurately controlled infusion systems have been important factors in the successes achieved by neonatologists.

As the prognosis for survival improves, so attention is being turned from the chest to the brain. The long-term outlook for pre-term infants ultimately depends to some extent on the avoidance of injury whether physical or chemical to the brain during birth and the neonatal period. Although the link between neonatal problems and brain injury was long recognized by pathologists, it was not until imaging techniques suitable for use in living infants were developed that the very high incidence of brain injury from haemorrhage and ischaemia (inadequate blood supply) was appreciated. As computerized axial tomography (an X-ray technique which reveals far more than a 'straight' X-ray) and, later, portable ultrasound scanners have become widely used the factors and events antecedent to brain injury have become better understood.

A major factor of most of these brain lesions is probably abnormal cerebral blood flow, either too much or too little, and a relative lack of appropriate control of the circulation. Because the methods used to measure the cerebral circulation in the adult were not considered safe in small babies a number of attempts at non-invasive measurement were made in the 1970s, but these were only partly successful. Improvements in the technology of Doppler ultrasound have resulted in a large increase in the number of reports about the cerebral circulation in sick infants, but the techniques as yet can at best measure only the velocity rather than the volume flow of the cerebral circulation. A newer technique shows great promise and uses the absorption of infra-red light transmitted across the infant's brain to gain information about the cerebral perfusion and state of cerebral oxygenation. Another technique, magnetic resonance spectroscopy (an electro–magnetic form of 'imaging'), has also been used to measure the state of energy metabolism within the brain following asphyxia and haemorrhage. Although none of these techniques is likely to find its way into daily use in every new-born unit in the land, the information provided by them should enable the treatment of the sick new-born infant in future to be based more and more on scientifically validatable principles rather than on empirical methods.

Later outcome

The significance of low birth-weight for the individual surviving child and his family is only revealed by long-term follow-up, and for the community can only be determined by true population-based surveys. The fact that babies less than 2.5 kg in weight at birth are of two main types, those born too early and those born too small, or a mixture of both was not generally appreciated until the 1950s, but has proved to be of importance in later outcome. The first national survey, the 1946 Maternity Survey, was initiated before the inception of the National Health Service (Douglas 1960). Other population-based surveys (with the birth-date of the infants sampled in brackets) came from Baltimore, USA (1952) (Wiener 1968), the British National Child Development Study (1958) (Fogelman 1983), the US Collaborative Perinatal Project (1959–1965) (Nelson and Ellenberg 1986), the Newcastle-upon-Tyne cohort from the surveys there of maternity and child development (1960–1962) (Neligan, Kolvin, Scott, and Garside 1976), and two northern provinces of Finland (1966) (Rantakallio and von Wendt 1985). Three other large studies deserve mention for their immense detail, though they were not true population surveys: a Medical Research Council cohort of consecutively admitted babies to 14 units in different parts of the UK (1951–1953) (McDonald 1967), an Edinburgh study (1953–1955) (Drillien 1964), in which assessments were carried out by a single investigator who gained valuable insights into the families concerned, and one from Vancouver (1959–1965) (Dunn 1986). The majority of these studies used infants of normal birth-weight for comparison (controls). Between them they confirmed that when mothers of low-birth-weight infants were compared to control mothers they were found more often to have a history of previous infertility, recurrent abortion, still births, or previous low birth-weight, and tended to have had less antenatal care but more complicated pregnancies. In addition they more often came from a background of socio–economic disadvantage, were more likely to be very young or above average age, to smoke more, and to be unmarried—all factors which also have importance for the postnatal environment of the child.

The surveys also confirmed that cerebral palsy, fits, mental retardation, educational subnormality, behaviour disorders, impaired perceptuomotor skills (appreciation of shape, form or order and control of muscular movement), school learning difficulties, varying degrees of visual and hearing impairment, and short stature were found approximately three- to five-times more commonly in low-birth-weight infants than in controls. Sequelae were most likely in those who had been ill in the neonatal period and the growth-retarded infants did less well than those normally grown at birth. The incidence of recorded impairments which together or singly gave rise to varying disabilities and handicap increased as birth-weight and gestational age decreased. But as these smallest babies—those less than 1.5 kg in weight—comprise only a little over 10 per cent of low-birth-weight births, which themselves account for only 6–7 per cent of all live births, low-birth-weight *per se* has never in the past been the major source of serious childhood disability. Thus if 70 per cent survive and 20 per cent of survivors are disabled, less than one in a thousand children will be disabled by this cause.

Most reports published since neonatal intensive care was more widely applied at the end of the 1960s and the 1970s have concentrated on the very low-birth-weight infant. Many have come from individual units practising the new technology, all of them dealing with highly selected populations. The majority have been optimistic in tone. There have been a few surveys of defined populations, though the children involved were mostly very young at the time of reporting. One exception is the Aberdeen survey of all infants of birth-weight 2.5 kg or less born in the one year between 1969 and 1970, who were tested at ten years (Illsley and Mitchell 1984). There was neurological abnormality in 9 per cent of the low-birth-weight sample and 0.7 per cent of normal birth-weight controls. The low-birth-weight group scored less well on intelligence tests, but, as in the 1946 survey, although careful matching with control families had been undertaken on socio-economic grounds at birth, the socio-cultural background of the low-birth-weight families later turned out to be poorer in many subtle ways.

Studies from an urban South Ontario county in Canada revealed that mortality had been substantially reduced for babies weighing 0.5–1.5 kg at birth during the years 1973–1977 compared to the pre-intensive care years, 1964–1969, but among survivors there had been no change in percentage morbidity (Horwood, Boyle, Torrance, and Sinclair 1982). Neurological impairments—cerebral palsy, hydrocephalus, microcephaly (abnormally small brain), blindness, deafness, and mental retardation—occurred in 17 per cent of those babies born during 1973-1978 (Saigal, Rosenbaum, Stoskopf, and Milner 1982). Later comparison of babies weighing up to 1 kg at birth reported that 55 per cent and 53 per cent of survivors were considered functionally handicapped in the 1973-1976 and 1977-1980 groups respectively, but the actual number of affected children in the later period, though small in absolute numbers, was double that of the earlier period because there were more survivors (Saigal, Rosenbaum, Stoskopf, and Sinclair 1984).

The prevalence of cerebral palsy and severe educational sub-normality among children in a Medical Research Council study conducted in 1950 of 14 UK units was compared with that among school-age children of the same birth-weight born in the South East Thames region of London in 1970, 1971, and 1973 (Alberman, Benson, and McDonald 1982). Prevalence was found to be lower for one or both defects in the later years, partly due to a fall in the incidence of births of very short gestation and a reduction of risk in the immature births. The lessened risk, however, was counterbalanced by the increased survival so that there was little alteration in the overall numbers. Among Wolverhampton infants weighing less than 1.5 kg at birth and born in the period 1975-1979, 49 per cent of 51 school-age survivors were performing poorly at school, compared with sibling (brother and sister) controls (Lloyd 1984). If this finding is confirmed in a larger survey it might be at odds with the conclusions drawn from the Aberdeen study that it is the unfavourable social environment which largely accounts for the disadvantage of being low birth-weight. In five adjacent districts of the Mersey region, over 1000 surviving babies born in 1979-1981 and weighing 2 kg or less at birth were assessed by a single doctor at pre-school age (Powell, Pharoah, and Cooke 1986). When the cohort was compared with some of the earlier population surveys mentioned above the proportion of babies surviving without major impairment was judged to have increased significantly. However, the risk of surviving with any impairment had not changed enough for a significant difference to be obvious.

It is clear that continuing population studies will be needed to assess the extent to which the number of surviving low-birth-weight infants with disability is static or increasing. As survival at all birth-weights accelerates, the proportion of survivors with disabilities will have to fall considerably if actual numbers of disabled children in the community are not to increase. The inference from several of the studies recorded here must be that numbers are increasing. The adequate ascertainment of these children at 2-3 years of age has still to be considered far from complete, however, and comparing pre-school children with children of school age who have had detailed and standardized testing is misleading. Further, among infants of very low birth-weight, impairments are subtly changing. None of those recorded 20-30 years ago have disappeared although retinopathy of prematurity with resultant blindness became very uncommon in the late 1950s and 1960s. In the USA, however, over 4000 infants have been blinded so far in a second 'epidemic' of retrolental fibroplasia compared with over 7000 in the 1940s. The birth-weight of the majority of these blind infants is below 1.0 kg, whereas in the 1940s numbers of such infants surviving were negligible and those weighing 1.0-1.5 kg were mostly involved. Accurate recent figures for retinopathy of prematurity in this country are not available.

There are also changes in the pattern of residual neurological disability. Thirty to forty years ago low birth-weight infants developing cerebral palsy usually had spastic diplegia, in which the legs were more involved than the arms and in which the intelligence was often in the normal range. Now at least one regional study has shown an increase in more complex and disabling forms of residual cerebral palsy, with mental subnormality. A proportion of young survivors now too have shunted post-haemorrhagic hydrocephalus (i.e. hydrocephalus developing as a result of bleeding into the cerebral ventricles, which is common in very low-birth-weight infants, and treated by a shunt).

Mechanical ventilation, which undoubtedly allows many seriously ill infants to survive, can also cause a form of lung damage— bronchopulmonary dysplasia—in the most immature infants and in those ventilated for long periods. It may leave the children oxygen dependent and breathless and at increased risk from respiratory infection in the first six months of life. Full recovery of normal pulmonary function as assessed by detailed testing is unlikely, though there is a significant decrease of symptoms towards the end of the first year.

Total parenteral nutrition, a technique which allows babies to be fed entirely intravenously, has been associated with prolonged jaundice and increased infection rates in some infants, and, while most appear to recover completely, few long-term studies of the effect of this procedure, particularly on liver function, are available. Recently the possibility of cerebral injury from high levels of phenylalanine and other amino acids in infants receiving intravenous nutrition has been raised.

A number of infants have noticeable skin scarring following intravenous infusions when fluid has accidentally leaked into fragile subcutaneous tissues. Some such scars, including others on the chest from tubes inserted to drain free air from the chest cavity following lung rupture (pneumothorax), are very unsightly and may cause personal distress as the scars grow in size with the growth of the individual.

The number of X-rays taken of small ill babies receiving intensive care between the time of their pre-term birth and their expected date of delivery has increased considerably. It will be many years before any harmful effects can be detected.

Other forms of treatment, or new diagnostic methods, while apparently safe in the short term, need very long-term surveillance to be pronounced completely safe. Even the constantly lit, often very noisy ambience of the intensive care unit may have as yet unrecognized hazards.

One rather unique cohort of infants (0.501–1.5 kg in weight) born in Mansfield and district during the years 1963–1971 before neonatal mortality began to decrease considerably was reported in 1980 (Steiner, Sanders, Phillips, and Maddock 1980). Medical care there had been of a deliberately non-interventionist nature and standards of nursing care and record keeping were stated to be high. The outcome regarding survival, disability, and intelligence at school age compared favourably with that reported by units undertaking intensive care during the same period.

A controlled trial of what was called intensive care (although it did not include mechanical ventilation) between 1966 and 1970 in an Australian neonatal unit for infants weighing 1.0–1.5 kg at birth showed a significantly increased survival for those treated intensively, but also significantly more disabled children at eight years of age (Kitchen, Rickards, Ryan, McDougall, Billson, Keir, and Naylor 1979).

None of these follow-up surveys has found low-birth-weight infants as a group to be the equal of their normal birth-weight peers. The majority, however, who belong to the higher birth-weights will be indistinguishable from normal in later life, except on very detailed testing, and sometimes on account of small stature. The first year of life is often the most testing for the families of these infants. Apart from the anxieties faced in the neonatal period and weeks beyond until discharge, low-birth-weight children may need further admissions to hospital, usually because of respiratory infections. The risk of sudden, unexpected death, and of child abuse, is also greatest during this year. A proportion of such children, although apparently normal, will have learning difficulties at school, which may, however, be identified by appropriate screening tests before school entry. These learning difficulties, if not identified for remedial help, may be serious enough to lead to academic failure, often with attendant behaviour problems. The academic achievement of children depends to some extent on parental interest and encouragement; but several surveys have shown that many families of low-birth-weight children fail to provide the necessary stimulating atmosphere.

Thus among all children a small number of low-birth-weight children, derived mostly from the 5 per cent who weigh less than 1.25 kg at birth, will face significant functional disability. The extent to which this becomes a handicap often depends upon the resources of the family. Some families are strengthened by disability but others are shattered by it. For those who find difficulty in coping, the help they receive from the community is often crucial. In many areas this support is seriously underprovided, of poor quality, and seldom continues into adult life.

Resuscitation of the asphyxiated new-born

There is no generally agreed definition of birth asphyxia, but failure to establish spontaneous breathing within two minutes of delivery occurs in up to 15 per cent of all births and is significantly more likely to occur in infants of low birth-weight, in multiple pregnancy, in infants born by Caesarean section, and following breech delivery or complex forceps delivery. The role of active resuscitation at birth is never likely to be defined by a controlled trial. That resuscitation has some role in lowering mortality cannot be doubted, as there are cases on record in which no heart beat or respiratory gasp was detected at birth yet prompt resuscitation converted these apparent still births to live births. Further, such children, providing there was no antecedent severe fetal distress, often turn out to be apparently normal. Prompt and active resuscitation for infants weighing between 1 and 2 kg at birth was associated with a 20 per cent reduction in mortality from hyaline membrane disease in Newcastle-upon-Tyne during 1971–1976 compared to an earlier period, 1960–1967, when active resuscitation was not carried out. No other identifiable changes in management had occurred between the two time periods.

Birth asphyxia is frequently accompanied by a serious fall in body temperature. Prevention of this fall has been shown for many years to be associated with better survival rates, at least in low-birth-weight infants.

Although intrapartum asphyxia (i.e. during delivery) may be responsible for some cases of severe mental retardation and cerebral palsy, a sifting of all the epidemiological evidence suggests that it is certainly not the major cause. More than 75 per cent of cases of severe mental retardation unassociated with cerebral palsy (IQ less than 50) are prenatally determined. A recent re-analysis of data from the US Collaborative Perinatal Project suggests a relatively minor role for intrapartum factors in accounting for cerebral palsy. Thus active resuscitation at birth will not necessarily prevent mental retardation or cerebral palsy from occurring, although it may. Data from defined populations in Sweden and northern England suggest a rise in the prevalence of cerebral palsy from the mid-1960s to the mid-1970s, involving all birth-weights in Sweden but only those over 2.5 kg in England. This might be interpreted as increased survival of prenatally determined cerebral palsy through improved resuscitation and falling mortality rates, but there is no positive proof. It could equally be argued, again without proof, that but for active resuscitative measures some infants to whom these are applied and who develop normally would otherwise have suffered from cerebral palsy and that in consequence the rise in the incidence of cerebral palsy but for the resuscitative measures would have been even higher.

Resuscitation and viability

Resuscitation of new-born babies when based on sound physio-logical principles is a very effective form of medical treatment which does not cost very much to carry out. Nevertheless it represents the start of intensive care of the new-born in whom, as is often the case with pre-term infants, the problems at birth continue into the neonatal period. Some babies despite the most enthusiastic and capable management will not eventually survive or will survive with some disability. Much the same problem exists with starting intensive care in adults, but this is rarely held as a reason for not trying in the first place. The resuscitation of new-born babies is not a particularly 'high-tech' affair, and is most often carried out in the middle of the night by junior staff, who, although quite capable of the procedures required, often will not have the longer term experience on which rapid decisions about the appropriateness of resuscitation in individual cases is best based. Often most concern is expressed about the resuscitation of the extremely pre-term infant who might survive with disability or die after a prolonged period of intensive care.

In practice the very pre-term infant, apart from being a rare creature, is very likely to make his own decision about survival despite the efforts of his attendants. A much greater disaster is the term infant who just survives after prolonged attempts at resuscitation and does so, often with minimal after-care, to live a severely disabled life. Fear of outcome may engender in some attendants reluctance to even attempt resuscitation in the very pre-term infant. It is necessary, however, to appreciate that during intensive care the time may come when further efforts are unlikely to achieve much or improve ultimate prognosis, and extraordinary means of care should be stopped. Such decisions are not easy to make and may involve a degree of heart-searching, but are better made in the light of the fullest information available than in haste at the moment of birth. Wider public discussion and involvement in such issues, rather than legislation and ill-informed recrimination, is necessary to help doctors to make correct decisions in these difficult circumstances.

The cost of neonatal care

In an ideal world, the cost of medical and nursing care would not be a factor in determining care for babies. But the rapidly rising costs and increasingly complex technologies make some form of economic assessment essential, even if it is only to justify the current level of expenditure. Costing studies are very complicated and only two have been published in the UK. North American studies are available, but difficult to extrapolate to the situation here because of differences in the methods of providing and paying for health care.

The cost of care must be balanced against the benefits likely to be achieved from giving that care. Fewer larger babies require intensive care, and those that do generally need it for a relatively short period. Outcome with a few exceptions is good. The balance of costs against benefits weighs in favour of intensive care. For the very small infant the situation is different. Greater costs, and a higher likelihood of long-term disability, make the balance of cost and benefit less favourable. A number of North American studies have concluded that, overall, infants of below about 1 kg in weight cost so much that their economic contribution in life-time earnings does not on average meet their life-time medical costs. As a result restrictive policies for the institution of intensive care in tiny babies have been suggested. This approach is not very logical, as many paediatricians will be aware that most of the very small babies who survive do so with little intensive care with apparently normal outcome. The problems of generalizing were shown by a study from Liverpool (Sandhu, Stevenson, Cooke, and Pharoah 1986) which demonstrated that while the cost of intensive care did generally increase in smaller babies the correlation was largely an artefact produced by grouping the data into 100 g weight groups. Individual costing of infants' care resulted in virtually no correlation between cost of care and birth-weight. Other points arising from this study were that staff costs and hospital overheads were 60 per cent of total costs whereas equipment accounted for less than 5 per cent. In 1984 ventilator care cost £297 per day and high dependency care £138. The average cost of hospital intensive care for a survivor under 1.5 kg in weight was £4490 but there was a very wide variation in this.

Attempts to examine the cost–benefit ratio of neonatal intensive care in terms of quality adjusted life years gained (QUALYs) have been made. The long survival of neonatal patients after discharge and their good outcome acts in their favour in such an assessment. Neonatal intensive care ranks with renal transplantation in equivalent cost–benefit.

Examining the make-up of these costs it can be seen that the economies on equipment replacement and drugs that are usually suggested are the least likely to make a significant impact on the overall expenditure. Stopping care when the probability of a good outcome is low could reduce costs, but the problem is to assess accurately this probability and to decide what chance is too small to be worth taking. Ultimately real cost reduction can only come from reducing the number of infants being born who require such care. Whether in the long term the cost of the necessary health education, change of life-style, and economic circumstances needed to achieve this will be less than that of intensive care is difficult to assess, but it would be a better solution.

Conclusions and implications for the future

The care of new-born babies has come to occupy a steadily increasing proportion of paediatricians' time relative to the older child, and it is now one of the main paediatric specialities. Much of the time is spent on problems such as routine physical examination (screening), feeding difficulties, the many lesser illnesses, and advising mothers, which do not come within the realm of intensive care. During the 40 years or so of paediatric responsibility for the new-born infant, there has been a very great increase in awareness of developmental physiology, biochemistry, and pharmacology. At the beginning of this period even basic skills of care such as inserting a tube into the trachea (wind pipe) for resuscitation at birth had to be self-taught. Now young doctors and nurses have achieved experience in this and many other techniques used with tiny babies. Advances in electronic equipment have extended further the levels of care possible. These developments applied to seriously ill older infants and children have also benifited them. A better understanding of parental needs pervades most maternity and neonatal units now. Healthy babies 'room-in' with their mothers instead of being banished to nurseries for much of the day and all of the night. Parents of very ill babies are positively encouraged to be involved in their care instead of viewing them from behind glass screens for a few minutes a day. Explanations, progress reports, and emotional support are more readily forthcoming than ever before.

While neonatal mortality had been falling steadily since the beginning of the century, due more to social and demographic changes than to medical care, the rate of fall has accelerated since 1975 particularly for those babies of very low birth-weight. There is evidence from this country and abroad to suggest that the more general application of neonatal intensive care, fostered by a handful of units to begin with, together with the concerned interest and skill of obstetricians, is responsible for much of the new survival. Regional centres have been designated over much of the country, but there remains a shortage of nursing and medical personnel for the intensity of care presently practised. The surgical treatment of congenital malformations has widened in scope and is increasingly successful. The main preoccupations are still the same as those of 40 years ago: malformations, birth asphyxia, and low birth-weight.

Neonatal care has some impressive achievements, but there must always be some concern when intensive care is needed at the beginning of life. When intensive care was much less intensive than now, there was some evidence that, compared with routine care, intensive care increased survival but also disability. This may or may not be true now: for most low-birth-weight infants more effective intensive care may be producing better results, with more survivors and with no more, and probably less, disability. For the extremely small infant below 28 weeks of gestation, however, the application of increasingly intensive care may be producing diminishing returns, for the formidable problems imposed by the care itself now have to be added to the risk of those impairments always known to be more common in such infants. Many of the present treatments and diagnostic aids need to be proved safe in the long term. Commitment to long-term surveillance of the survivors of intensive care is a matter of national importance and needs to be encouraged.

It has been pointed out by others that the most skilled medical care cannot compensate for the results of socio-economic deprivation. The low-birth-weight rate is a pointer to national health, yet has remained unchanged for more than 30 years. If the number of children growing up in relative poverty is now increasing, we may expect the low-birth-weight rate to increase, with all the disadvantages to the survivors which that implies. Paediatricians caring for the new-born infant in the future must concern themselves not only with the medical problems of babies and their parents but also with the socio-economic factors which contribute to these problems.

References

Alberman, E., Benson, J., and McDonald, A. (1982). Cerebral palsy and severe educational subnormality in low-birthweight children: a comparison of births in 1951–53 and 1970–73. *Lancet* **1**, pp. 606–8.

Douglas, J. W. B. (1960). 'Premature' children at primary schools. *British Medical Journal* **1**, pp. 1008–13.

Drillien, C. M. (1964). *The growth and development of the prematurely born infant.* E & S Livingstone, Edinburgh.

Dunn, H. G. (ed.) (1986). *Sequelae of low birthweight: the Vancouver study.* Clinics in Developmental Medicine no. 95/96. Blackwell Scientific Publications, Oxford.

Fogelman, K. (ed.) (1983). *Growing up in Great Britain. Papers from the National Child Development Study.* Macmillan, London.

Horwood, S. P., Boyle, M. H., Torrance, G. W., and Sinclair, J. C. (1982). Mortality and morbidity of 500- to 1,499-gram birth weight infants live-born to residents of a defined geographic region before and after neonatal intensive care. *Pediatrics* **69**, pp. 613–20.

Illsley, R. and Mitchell, R. G. (Eds.) (1984). *Low birth weight: a medical, psychological and social study.* John Wiley, Chichester.

Kitchen, W. H., Rickards, A., Ryan, M. M., McDougall, A. B., Billson, F. A., Keir, E. H., and Naylor, F. D. (1979). A longitudinal study of very-low-birthweight infants. II: Results of controlled trial of intensive care and incidence of handicaps. *Developmental Medicine and Child Neurology* **21**, pp. 582–9.

Lloyd, B. W. (1984). Outcome of very-low-birthweight babies from Wolverhampton. *Lancet* **2**, pp. 739–41.

Macartney, F. J., Taylor, J. F. N., Graham, G. R., de Leval, M., and Stark, J. (1980). The fate of survivors of cardiac surgery in infancy. *Circulation* **62**, pp. 80–91.

McDonald, A. (1967). *Children of very low birth weight.* MEIU research monograph no. 1. Heinemann Medical Books, London.

Macfarlane, A. and Mugford M. (1984) *Birth Counts. Statistics of pregnancy and childbirth.* HMSO, London.

Neligan, G. A., Kolvin, I., Scott, D. M., and Garside, R. F. (1976). *Born too soon or born too small.* Clinics in Developmental Medicine no. 61. Heinemann Medical Books, London.

Nelson, K. B. and Ellenberg, J. H. (1986). Antecedents of cerebral palsy. Multivariate analysis of risk. *New England Journal of Medicine* **315**, pp. 81–6.

Pharoah, P. O. D. and Alberman, E. D. (1981). Mortality of low birthweight infants in England and Wales 1953–79. *Archives of Disease in Childhood* **56**, pp. 86–9.

Powell, T. G., Pharoah, P. O. D., and Cooke, R. W. I. (1986). Survival and morbidity in a geographically defined population of low-birthweight infants. *Lancet* **1**, pp. 539–43.

Rantakallio, P. and von Wendt, L. (1985). Prognosis for low-birthweight infants up to the age of 14: a population study. *Developmental Medicine and Child Neurology* **27**, pp. 655–63.

Saigal, S., Rosenbaum, P., Stoskopf, B., and Milner, R. (1982). Follow-up of infants 501–1500 gm birth-weight delivered to residents of a geographically defined region with perinatal intensive care facilities. *Journal of Pediatrics* **100**, pp. 606–13.

Saigal, S., Rosenbaum, P., Stoskopf, B., and Sinclair, J. C. (1984). Outcome in infants 501 to 1000 gm birth–weight delivered to residents of the McMaster Health Region. *Journal of Pediatrics* **105**, pp. 969–76.

Sandhu, B., Stevenson, R. C., Cooke, R. W. I., and Pharoah, P. O. D. (1986). Cost of neonatal intensive care for very-low-birthweight infants. *Lancet* **1**, pp. 600–3.

Steiner, E. S., Sanders, E. M., Phillips, E. C. K., and Maddock, C. R. (1980). Very-low-birth-weight children at school age: comparison of neonatal management methods. *British Medical Journal* **281**, pp. 1237–40.

Weiner, G. (1968). Scholastic achievement at age 12–13 of prematurely born children. *Journal of Special Education* **2**, pp. 237–50.

4

The reality of handicap

MARTIN C. O. BAX, ROGER J. ROBINSON,
and ANN GATH

Introduction

The World Health Organization has usefully made the distinction between: an *impairment*, which describes a pathological process such as spina bifida; a *disability*, which is the consequence of that impairment (this might be someone without an arm who lacks bi-manual activity); and a *handicap*, which is the social consequence of impairment or disability—reflecting the way an individual responds to his impairment and dysfunction. A person who has had an amputation resulting from an accident and has an appropriate prosthesis (artificial limb) may not be worried by his disability and could be described as not being handicapped; an individual with no disability but an impairment such as a disfiguring port-wine stain of the face may be so ashamed of this disfigurement that he is not prepared to go out during the day, may fail to obtain a job, and become socially isolated and handicapped. Handicap is to some extent in the eye of the beholder. A person with muscular dystrophy recently reported that he was not handicapped, although he was wheel-chair bound, but told how, stuck at the bottom of a lift, he was too weak in the arms to reach up to press the buttons. Most people would feel that such an individual was handicapped.

For the young child the judgement that he is handicapped is not one he makes himself but one that is made by those around him. Later, handicap may exist at certain times but not at others. A child with Down's syndrome but of fair intelligence may do quite well in ordinary school and so be judged non-handicapped when he is seven, eight, or nine years old, but by the time of puberty lack of social skills may mean that he is much more handicapped.

Thus initially parents and surrounding professionals make the decision that a child is handicapped. Later the child may or may not feel that he is handicapped. The present chapter considers people who in early life are judged by parents and professionals alike as being handicapped, but recognizes that the individual's own view of self is important once the age of puberty is reached.

How many children are handicapped?

Given that handicap is a social condition it is not surprising that it is difficult to say precisely how many handicapped children there are in the community. Often we lack reliable, up-to-date data on the numbers with any particular medical diagnosis. The Warnock Report (1978) suggested that as many as one in five schoolchildren might at some time have special needs beyond those met routinely in schools. Not all children with perhaps a temporary difficulty are really handicapped and it seems more reasonable to consider particularly the 1 or 2 per cent of children with severe handicap who will attend District Handicap Teams. The largest group will be the mentally handicapped, among whom Down's syndrome is the commonest diagnosis, and next the physically handicapped, including children with cerebral palsy, muscular dystrophy, and spina bifida, three conditions which make up two-thirds of the physically handicapped population. The sensory handicaps—significant visual or hearing problems—are less common. Categories of handicap may of course overlap; thus a child may be mentally retarded, have cerebral palsy, a visual handicap, and in addition behaviour problems. It was for this reason that the Warnock Committee abandoned the categories of handicap, but instead talked about children with special needs. The disadvantages of this are discussed later. Some details of the numbers of children with particular diagnoses are given below.

The disorders

There are a large number of chronically handicapping disorders in childhood. Our main emphasis is on those causing chronic neurological impairment since these cause the greatest burden to the largest number of families. We also mention briefly some of the important non-neurological disorders.

Some of the headings used are diagnoses in the ordinary medical sense—well-defined disorders which have a recognized cause with similar or identical features in all patients suffering from them. Others, numerically the most important, are not diagnoses in this sense, but descriptions of functional disturbances which vary widely in cause, severity, and clinical features. The distinction between these two categories is important, not just to enable professionals to think clearly about the terms they use, but also to help parents understand the sort of evaluating process their child will undergo when, for example, he is referred to a Child Development Centre. There, questions will be asked about the history, and the child will be examined (including watching his performance at various tasks) in order to try to answer two different kinds of question. The first concerns causation or aetiology: is the cause of the child's disability known or can it be discovered? Special investigations such as chromosome analysis and brain scanning may help to provide an answer but in many chronic neurological diseases of childhood the fundamental cause cannot be found. The second kind of question concerns the child's functioning—what are his skills and attainments and what difficulties does he have compared with other children of the same age? Further assessments, using standardized quantitative tests, may be done by psychologists, speech therapists, or oc-cupational therapists. Motor function may be examined in more detail by a physiotherapist. It is this functional assessment, rather than the search for a cause, which will usually lead to plans for helping the child. If parents do not understand the distinction between these two kinds of question—because the professionals do not explain their purpose—they may finish the consultation feeling confused. They may, for example, feel that because a medical diagnosis has not been made, it is not possible to make plans to help the child. The question 'Is he brain-damaged?' often raises this sort of confusion. It may mean either, 'Does he have some sign of physical damage to the brain, seen for instance on the brain scan?' or 'Does he have the pattern of difficulty in learning and behaviour which psychologists have sometimes called brain damage?'

Mental handicap

Of all the chronic disorders of childhood, mental retardation is the most important both because of its commonness and because of the burden it imposes on the family. Mental retardation may be defined in terms of measured intelligence (the psychometric defin-ition) or of the individual's ability to cope with education and later with independent living (the social definition). The social definition is generally more useful practically, and usually identifies a smaller number of people as mentally retarded than the psychometric definition. The latter is useful in research, and also in indicating the variations in severity of mental retardation. A useful subdivision in psychometric terms is into three grades.

Categories and incidence of mental retardation   The *mildly mentally retarded* have intelligence quotients (IQs) (IQ represents mental age expressed as a percentage of actual age) between about 50 and 70. They are slower than their peers in learning at school and need special educational help. However, when they reach adult life they will mostly integrate into the ordinary community and lead independent lives. Mild mental retardation affects between 1 and 3 per cent of the population.

The *severely mentally retarded* have IQs below 50. Their educational ability is much more limited (though it is important not to underestimate it, and many of these children achieve far more nowadays with pre-school learning programmes and a more optimistic attitude to their educational potential). In adult life they will usually need a sheltered environment and will not be wholly independent.

It has become customary to recognize simply these two grades of mental retardation—mild and severe—but it is useful to identify a third group—the *profoundly mentally retarded*—at the lower end of the severe group. These individuals have IQs too low to measure meaningfully, are not able to benefit from formal education in the ordinary sense, need special education with an emphasis on self-care and other skills of daily living, and will continue to need a great deal of care and attention throughout their lives. They will often have additional disabilities such as cerebral palsy and epilepsy. Their life expectancy is likely to be shortened, but even the most profoundly handicapped given good care at home will often reach adult life. This knowledge is of great importance to parents, who have anxieties as to what will happen to their handicapped offspring when they are old or have died. Severe and profound mental retardation affect about 0.3 per cent of the population.

Causes of mental handicap   The causes of mental handicap are very varied, and include a large number of genetic and environmental factors. In many mentally retarded children it is not possible to identify the cause, even after careful study of the history, detailed examination, and use of all modern diagnostic techniques including brain scanning. Parents often find the inability of doctors to find the cause of their child's disability hard to understand. Finding the cause is unlikely to alter management, but it does help parents' understanding of the problem, may give a clearer indication of the risks to future children of that couple, and, of course, knowing the cause of a disorder is the first step towards prevention.

Mild mental retardation is strongly related to social class and is much commoner among the socially disadvantaged in whom it is usually the result of a combination of genetic and environmental factors, each individually too small to be identified. There has been much controversy about the relative importance of genetic and environmental factors, but there is good evidence that both are important. The most helpful approach to prevention is probably social and educational with the object of removing inequalities in environment, education, and opportunity.

Mental retardation may also be the result of a single factor which has damaged the brain or interfered with its development. In general these single identifiable factors are likely to cause severe retardation but this is only a rough generalization and some abnormalities of the sex chromosomes, for example, may cause relatively mild retardation. Chromosome abnormalities are among the most important identifiable causes. Down's syndrome due to an extra chromosome 21 (the chromosomes, 46 in number, are numbered in pairs from one to 22, and there are also two sex chromosomes, boys having an X and a Y chromosome and girls two X chromosomes) is the best known example. It affects approximately one child in 600, and accounts for about one-third of severe retardation. The major recent advance in this field has been the discovery of the 'fragile X' chromosome (not an alteration in the number of chromosomes but a detectable abnormality in the X chromosome). This may prove to be almost as common a cause of mental retardation as Down's syndrome. It affects either sex, although originally thought to be confined to boys. Chromosome analysis is time-consuming and expensive, and it is not at present possible to carry it out on all mentally retarded people.

Mental retardation may be the result of other genetically determined syndromes, some of which also result in 'dysmorphism' (recognizable patterns of malformation) and some in inborn errors of metabolism. It may also result from adverse factors affecting the developing embryo or fetus—known examples being maternal infections such as rubella (German measles), cytomegalovirus infection (a virus which can be transmitted from mother to fetus during pregnancy and damage the fetus), toxoplasmosis (a protozoon which can be transferred from mother to fetus), herpes, and maternal toxins such as alcohol in excessive amounts. Some prenatal factors remain unrecognized and constitute a major cause of mental retardation.

Disorders or accidents in the perinatal period (see Chapter 3) or at later stages in infancy or childhood can cause brain damage. Severe head injury, either accidental or non-accidental, acute brain disorders such as encephalitis, or severe interference with the oxygen supply to the brain—for example, from asphyxia in fires, drowning accidents, and complications of difficult anaesthesia or cardiac surgery—come into this category. Perinatal and postnatal causes probably account for less than one-third of severe mental retardation, and in these cases the handicap is often complex, including cerebral palsy and/or epilepsy. Medical intervention is more likely to be effective in prevention where there is a single identifiable cause: antenatal diagnosis with termination of pregnancy may be one solution, and optimum management of perinatal and postnatal causes of retardation such as asphyxia (lack of oxygen) may mitigate their brain-damaging effects.

Cerebral palsy

Cerebral palsy is a disorder of great practical and social importance, but it is not an easy one to define or explain. Patients with cerebral palsy do not all have the same problems or disabilities—the term covers a number of clinical syndromes, differing widely in their causes, neurological features, and the degree of handicap they cause. The lay term for people with cerebral palsy is 'spastics', though medically the term spastic is reserved for one particular variety of cerebral palsy.

Cerebral palsy has been defined as 'a persistent but not unchanging disorder of movement or posture due to a non-progressive defect or lesion of the immature brain'. This definition says three important things about children with cerebral palsy. First, they have a motor disorder ('movement and posture'); however, factors which damage the immature brain will seldom be so selective that they affect motor areas alone, and other associated disorders such as mental handicap, seizures, and problems of vision and/or hearing are common. If mental handicap is severe it will usually be the most important practical problem.

Second, the definition indicates that the brain abnormality dates from the period of brain development ('immature brain'). It may therefore arise during intra-uterine life, in the perinatal period, or in infancy or early childhood (usually taken to mean before age five).

Third, the brain disorder is non-progressive. The diagnosis therefore excludes degenerative brain disorders, tumours, and progressive hydrocephalus, even though these may produce very similar neurological problems. (The additional problems faced by the child and the family in the case of tumours and degenerative diseases are those of a disorder which is not only handicapping but may also be getting progressively worse and have a fatal outcome. Several different kinds of brain tumour occur in children, and some may be treated successfully by surgery, radiotherapy, or chemotherapy. The degenerative diseases, on the other hand, are a group of rare genetically determined metabolic disorders, for the great majority of which there is so far no treatment.)

Causes of cerebral palsy　There are many possible causes of cerebral palsy, since a large number of factors may damage the brain during development. It has been customary to group these causes according to when they operate. *Prenatal factors* account for an important proportion of cerebral palsy, but most cerebral palsy of prenatal origin is of unknown cause. Intra-uterine infections account for a very small proportion, as do chromosome abnormalities and other genetically determined disorders (see Chapter 2).

Perinatal factors (late in pregnancy, at delivery, and in the early days of life) are more easily recognized and have generally been assumed to account for at least half of all cerebral palsy. There is, however, some doubt as to whether a perinatal abnormality—such as birth asphyxia—occurring in a baby who subsequently proves to have cerebral palsy is necessarily the cause of the cerebral palsy: the baby may have been asphyxiated (failed to breathe) because there was an inherent brain abnormality disturbing the cerebral control of respiration.

Perinatal factors include birth trauma (though modern obstetric management has made this much less common) and hypoxia (shortage of oxygen supply to the brain) during labour, at birth, or in the early neonatal period. Neonatal jaundice used to be an important cause of a particular form of cerebral palsy, kernicterus. This has virtually disappeared because phototherapy and exchange transfusions (replacing the baby's blood with transfused blood) have made severe neonatal jaundice avoidable, and rhesus incompatibility, one of the main causes of severe neonatal jaundice, can now be prevented in most cases. Infants born prematurely are at considerably increased risk of developing cerebral palsy. They are more prone to the perinatal disorders already listed above but their excess of cerebral palsy does not seem to be fully accounted for in this way. Ultrasound studies of the brain of the prematurely born infant have shown a high frequency of two abnormalities which are associated with later cerebral palsy—intraventricular cerebral haemorrhage (bleeding into the cerebral ventricles, the cavities in the centre of the normal brain) and periventricular leucomalacia (softening of the area round the ventricles). They are probably due to interference with the cerebral circulation in premature infants.

Postnatal causes of cerebral palsy include many of the aetiologies listed above as well as strokes due to interference with the blood supply to the brain. They are less common, and account for about ten per cent of cases of cerebral palsy.

Types of cerebral palsy   For over a hundred years, attempts, none wholly successful, have been made to classify cerebral palsy into different types according to the nature of the motor disorder. Famous names such as Osler, Freud, and Little have been among those who tried to achieve a workable and rational classification. There are good reasons for making this attempt. First, patients suffering from cerebral palsy vary so greatly in their clinical features and disabilities that the description 'cerebral palsy' is almost meaningless without some further amplification. Second, it might be hoped that since cerebral palsy has many possible causes, and different types, a correlation might be found between particular types and particular causes, which would improve understanding of both. Such correlations, however, have only been found to a very limited extent. Third, the paediatrician or neurologist hopes that a classification will identify particular syndromes with constant features and a definable natural history, so that he can talk more sensibly to the parents about the future. Finally, the physical medicine specialist, physiotherapist, or orthopaediac surgeon may hope that classifying the motor disorder in a child will enable him to decide what forms of management will be most helpful. The following classification of cerebral palsy is practical and has proved clinically useful.

Spastic forms of cerebral palsy are those in which muscle tone and reflexes are increased. They can be subdivided into hemiplegia, affecting one side of the body; diplegia, affecting both sides, but the arms less than the legs; and quadriplegia, affecting all four limbs as well as the muscles used in feeding and speech.

Dystonic forms are those in which muscle tone is abnormal and variable, and differs from spasticity in that there may also be involuntary writhing (choreo-athetoid) movements.

Ataxic forms have mainly cerebellar signs—incoordination of voluntary movement.

In *hypotonic or atonic forms* there is general reduction in muscle tone. Some of these children will later develop signs of one of the other types of cerebral palsy, and some because of their associated mental status are probably better regarded as cases of severe mental retardation. The validity of including this term in the classification is doubtful.

Mixed types are those which share the features of more than one of the above types. This group is comparatively large—at least one-quarter of all cases.

It has to be admitted that such classifications are not wholly successful. Experienced doctors do not always agree on the class to which a patient belongs, and the purposes of classification as set out above have only been achieved to a limited extent.

The motor disorder in cerebral palsy not only leads to difficulties in movement, but often also to *contractures and deformities* of the trunk and limbs. Trying to prevent these problems, and treating them when they happen, is a team effort on the part of physiotherapists, orthopaedic surgeons, and other experts in the use of aids and appliances. The motor disorder may impair the patient's ability to communicate, and a small but very important group are those with relatively normal intelligence but a profound motor disorder, which makes speech impossible, and severely limits voluntary movements of the limbs. The intellectual ability of such children may not be recognized and therefore neglected to their severe disadvantage. Microcomputer technology has an increasing amount to offer these patients by providing alternative means of communication and expression.

Cerebral palsy is a persisting disorder, and it is important that the comprehensive services provided in childhood, to which schools for the physically handicapped contribute, should continue into adult life.

While perinatal factors are important in causing cerebral palsy, great advances have been made in managing these in recent years (Chapter 3). At the same time better perinatal care has increased the chances of survival of the smallest and sickest premature infants who are those with the greatest risk of developing cerebral palsy. The net result of these effects—whether cerebral palsy overall is occurring more or less frequently, and whether there is a change in pattern to low-birth-weight-related types—is a matter of great importance.

Spina bifida and hydrocephalus

Spina bifida is the commonest important malformation of the central nervous system causing chronic handicap. Its incidence varies in different parts of the world, and within different areas of the UK, being lowest in the south-east. There has been a marked fall in incidence over the past 20 years, only partly accounted for by the preventive measures described in Chapter 2. The present incidence is about one per 1000 births.

Spina bifida is due to a defect in closure of the neural tube during early intra-uterine life. The child is born with a sac over part of the spine. This contains membranes and usually malformed spinal cord. Several problems result. The sac may leak fluid and become infected, resulting in meningitis or ventriculitis (an infection inside the brain). The abnormality of the spinal cord is likely to cause weakness of the lower limbs, which may also lead to deformities and to impairment of bladder control. The kidneys may be seriously damaged. There is usually a hidden malformation at the junction of the brain and spinal cord—the so-called Arnold-Chiari mal-formation—which causes hydrocephalus in a high proportion of these children. Untreated, this may lead to mental retardation, blindness, and spasticity, as well as to an excessively large head. Children with spina bifida may also have severe spinal deformity and they are liable to other complex chronic handicaps.

There have been great changes in the management of and attitude to this congenital disorder during the lifetime of the British Paediatric Association (BPA). Sixty years ago the only treatment that could be offered was skin closure over the sac. Unfortunately when this was done the hydrocephalus often became more severe. More effective treatment was possible with the development of shunt procedures for hydrocephalus in the late-1950s. This was followed by a period of enthusiasm for radical treatment of spina bifida, including early closure of the back, shunting for hydrocephalus if needed, and vigorous treatment of the lower limb and bladder problems. By the early 1970s, however, it was realized that children and adolescents who had had radical treatment were a very handicapped group. Efforts were therefore made to select for treatment, on the basis of neurological findings at birth, those likely to be less severely handicapped and to treat these. In the others, nature would be allowed to take its course in the expectation that they would die within a few months. Such a policy was acceptable to most, including parents. However, ethical doubts aside, not all the babies expected to die quickly did so, and in some the back closure happened naturally. This and lessened incidence of the disorder has led to doubt about the reliability of very early selection for treatment or non-treatment. The fallibility of very early decisions on what to do has led to a more expectant approach, since there is no good evidence of harm from taking time over this.

Hydrocephalus may occur without spina bifida, as an isolated malformation or as a result of blockage to the outflow of cerebrospinal fluid from the brain by infection or haemorrhage. The last is particularly common in very premature infants who survive. Shunt operations for hydrocephalus have greatly improved since the 1950s, and the ventriculo–peritoneal shunts now most widely employed do not have such frequent or serious complications as the previous procedures. Nevertheless, blockage or infection of the shunt are still fairly common, and frequently require replacement of the shunt system. Thus children with shunts for hydrocephalus often need further operations, and untreated or unsuccessfully treated hydrocephalus is still a serious disorder.

Seizures and epilepsy

Fits or seizures are a manifestation of abnormal electrical discharge in the brain. Epilepsy means a tendency to recurrent seizures.

Seizures are commoner in childhood than at any other time of life. About 5 per cent of children will have a fit at some time, and about 0.5 per cent of schoolchildren have a persisting tendency to fits at least for some period. The various types of seizure which occur in older children and adults, including the so-called *grand mal type*, with major convulsions, and the *petit mal type*, with momentary 'absences', also occur in children, but several varieties of fits only occur in children. These include the following:

Neonatal fits are due to a variety of causes such as birth trauma or asphyxia, infection, and metabolic or biochemical problems. Certain types of neonatal fit indicate severe brain disturbance or abnormality and carry a definite risk of the child having later handicap. Other types may be of little significance.

Infantile spasms (salaam attacks), a particular variety of fit occurring in infancy, have recognized as well as unknown causes and carry a very high risk of later mental or neurological handicap.

Febrile convulsions, fits precipitated by fever in children between the ages of six months and five years, are the commonest of all childhood seizures, and fortunately the most benign. They are only associated with a slightly increased risk of later epilepsy.

The types of seizure which occur in children, their frequency, and their severity vary so greatly that generalizations about the degree of handicap they can cause are unhelpful. At the mildest end of the range is the child who has just one or two febrile convulsions or one fit without fever. These children do not normally require any treatment and suffer no disability but the episodes of fits may cause great anxiety to the parents. At the most severe end of the range are children with fits occurring many times a day, and not susceptible to drug treatment. These children often have other handicaps, including mental handicap. Seizures may be a feature of a· great variety of neurological disorders in childhood, and another distinction which therefore has to be made is between the child in whom seizures are the main or only problem and the child in whom they are but one part of a complex neurological handicap.

In the child whose seizures are his main problem, the prospects for control of the fits, and for outgrowing them, are reasonably good. Anticonvulsant drugs play an important part in treatment— they will often keep the child free of fits altogether, or at least reduce their frequency to an acceptable level. There is also some debatable evidence that preventing fits with anticonvulsant treatment may reduce the later liability to fits, enabling drugs to be withdrawn. The usual policy in the child who has had a number of fits without fever is to try to stop the fits completely with drugs and to continue drug treatment for two to three years before gradually stopping it if the child remains free of fits.

Even if treatment is successful, the epileptic child is a cause of anxiety to his parents. The fits themselves, possible dangers to the child, the social effects, possible stigmatization, and the possible restriction of activities all concern them. In adolescence, if fits persist, the questions of driving a motor car and of employment become increasingly important.

Anticonvulsant drugs, the mainstay of treatment, may also be a source of concern, because of the long period over which they need to be taken. Drugs used most frequently in the past certainly had a number of unwanted effects, including some on behaviour and school performance. The currently favoured drugs have fewer unwanted effects, but such can occur and considerable care over dosage is always needed. Continuance of the fits is likely to have a much worse effect.

The small group of children who have very frequent fits uninfluenced by currently available drugs remain a serious problem. Treatment by diet or surgery is sometimes successful, but in some of these children it simply has to be accepted that their seizures cannot be controlled and their lives and those of their families have to be adjusted accordingly. In the last resort residential schooling may be necessary when family and social disturbances caused by the epilepsy are adversely affecting control of the epilepsy itself.

Problems of speech, language, learning, and communication
Problems of language and of learning often both affect the same child. They are disorders in which paediatricians have become concerned relatively recently in the lifetime of the BPA with the growth of 'developmental' paediatrics. They are developmental problems, in the sense that the child is slower than his peers in acquiring the skills of speech, reading, or writing. Occasionally the disorders arise later as a result of illness or injury.

In the early years about 3 per cent of children will be sufficiently slow in *speech development* to worry their parents. Most of these children will talk normally by school age but may then have difficulty in learning to read or write and may need extra help at school. Somewhat under 1 per cent of children have a more severe or persisting disorder in learning to speak or to understand language. There are a number of possible causes, including deafness (it is essential that the child's hearing should be tested accurately), mental retardation, disorders which interfere with movements of the lips, tongue, or palate, and a social environment which does not provide the normal stimulus to language development. There is also a group of children with 'specific language disorders' in whom none of these causative factors operate. They are usually boys, and there is often a history of slow speech development in the family.

Children with the more severe degrees of *language delay* need effective neurological evaluation and, where indicated, speech therapy (which increasingly uses the skills and cooperation of the parents to carry out the programme). They also benefit from being in a nursery group or language unit using one of the programmes designed to accelerate language development. A small minority— perhaps of the order of one per thousand children—have speech and language problems persisting into school age, and they have special educational needs, which may include special schooling. The child with communication difficulties may well become frustrated and emotionally disturbed. Anything which helps him to communicate will help, such as the use of sign language, which the parents can learn.

By school age around 10 per cent of children have difficulties in acquiring *basic educational skills*. This may be the result of general slowness in learning either from social or cultural factors or from limited ability. Where the child has a 'specific learning difficulty', i.e. much more difficulty than his peers in learning to read and write despite normal intelligence and adequate schooling, the term 'dyslexia' is sometimes applied although controversy surrounds the definition and terminology of this. There is general agreement, however, that some children do have 'specific reading retardation' and need extra educational help.

The role of the paediatrician in helping the child with learning difficulties is still a matter of debate. He plays an important role in diagnosis. Professionals who play the most important part in assessing these children and planning help for them are teachers and educational psychologists. Their professional roles are clarified in the 1981 Education Act, which also gives parents a proper place in making plans for their child. An important medical contribution to the assessment of these children lies in excluding disorders of vision and hearing and checking for any important physical or neurological abnormality—rarely found, but important not to miss. This medical assessment is best done in the first instance by the school doctor or an appropriately trained general practitioner, who may then refer the child to the paediatrician, paediatric neurologist, or child development centre if further diagnostic sorting-out is needed.

The help for the child with learning problems is essentially educational, not medical, and is best given in the child's school or as near to it as possible. Paediatricians have often acted as advocates for the child, to ensure that he gets the help he needs, but this should be less necessary as the 1981 Education Act becomes fully effective.

Infantile autism and other pervasive developmental disorders Infantile autism, also known as Kanner's syndrome, is a form of severe pervasive developmental disorder in which there is delay and disorder of development of speech and non-verbal communication with impairment of ability to make social relationships. The autistic child also commonly shows other striking disturbances of behaviour, such as avoidance of eye contact, desire for sameness, preoccupation with particular objects or activities, and ritualistic repetitive mannerisms. Although a few children with these features have relatively normal non-verbal intelligence, the majority function at a mentally retarded level. Infantile autism affects about two or three children per 10 000. A larger group show *some* of the features of autism. Some are severely retarded with little or no language, and another group, now referred to as Asperger's syndrome, may talk fluently and at length but still have great difficulty in understanding subtle verbal and non-verbal communication. Assessment of intelligence and social behaviour is difficult but essential in children with autistic features if their educational needs are to be met.

Disorders of vision and hearing

Children with disorders of the special senses—vision and hearing—are important special groups among the handicapped. Their care and teaching are very specialized, but the paediatrician will be involved in their early diagnosis and the planning of their care.

Mild degrees of *hearing loss* are very common in children and are usually due to 'glue ear'—the result of infection or catarrh. While there is still considerable uncertainty about the importance of this disorder, and the extent to which it may cause impairment of speech or learning, it undoubtedly contributes to both these problems. There is also doubt about the correct treatment, and whether in the long run the widespread surgical use of 'grommets' to aerate the middle ear will prove to be the correct management.

Severe degrees of hearing loss are much less common, affecting about one to two children per 1000. Early diagnosis is very important in order that treatment can begin before speech development has become seriously delayed. The best screening procedure is still debated, but clinical testing of hearing at age eight months is the main method of detection. The severely deaf child will require hearing aids—expert knowledge is needed to prescribe these correctly, and a good deal of skill and care to ensure that they are correctly used. Speech therapy and pre-school learning opportunities are essential. The deaf child will also need special educational help, which increasingly is given in a special unit attached to a normal school. There has been dispute for well over a century about the best ways of teaching severely deaf children to talk, but there is now fairly widespread acceptance that alternative methods of communication such as sign language are a help rather than a hindrance.

Blindness or severe visual impairment are less common than deafness, affecting about three children per 10 000. Most commonly blindness is part of a more widespread handicapping disorder, which may include cerebral palsy or mental retardation. However, there are a number of disorders of the eyes themselves or of the optic nerves which lead to blindness alone. The blind child, like the severely deaf one, needs early diagnosis, his parents need early advice on helping his development, usually given by a peripatetic teacher of the blind, and special schooling is usually essential.

Muscle diseases

The 'neuromuscular disorders' are a group of disorders which affect either the muscles themselves or the nerve supply to them from the spinal cord. The brain is usually unaffected so that these children are generally of normal intelligence. Apart from the different nature of the motor disorder, two particular features distinguish the problems of these children from those posed by cerebral palsy. First, most of these diseases are progressive: child and family have to cope with steadily increasing weakness and ultimately death from the disorder. Deterioration may be quick, as in acute spinal muscular atrophy, where the child seldom lives much beyond the age of one year, or extremely slow, as in the common (Duchenne) form of muscular dystrophy, where an affected boy may live till his early twenties. Second, most of these diseases are inherited and carry predictable and usually high (e.g. one in four) risks of recurrence in further children of the same parents. There is currently active research into the prenatal detection of muscular dystrophy.

The commonest of the neuromuscular disorders is Duchenne-type muscular dystrophy, which affects about one boy in 5000. The weakness generally first becomes apparent before school age. From the age of about eight it becomes obviously progressive, and usually these boys are unable to walk by about age 12 or 13. Some centres have recently kept boys walking much longer by very vigorous orthopaedic treatment and the use of light-weight splints, and have found this improves morale and well-being. The usual cause of death is failure of the respiratory muscles and consequent chest infection. A very controversial form of treatment is to prolong life at this stage by mechanical support of ventilation.

Non-neurological disorders

We are not attempting here to describe all the physical disorders which may lead to chronic handicap in childhood. There are a large number of such but the burden of handicap which many impose is less than that caused by the neurological disorders already described—because most of them are less prevalent, or less disabling, or more effective treatment is available. Thus *congenital heart disease* is one of the commoner important congenital malformations, affecting nearly one child per 1000. However, some forms do not require treatment, and the more severe forms are much less likely to cause lasting disability as they are being treated with increasing success by surgery. Antenatal prevention and non-surgical methods of treatment are recent advances likely to reduce further the burden of handicap from congenital heart disease.

The treatment of the child with *chronic kidney disease* is another success story, though here the treatment—either by dialysis or kidney transplant—is very demanding on the child and family, often over a long period. *Chronic rheumatic diseases,* especially chronic juvenile arthritis, and the more severe *orthopaedic disorders,* also cause severe physical handicap in a number of children. They may require prolonged management regimens and may be attended by the social and psychological problems associated with reduced mobility.

Two further specific physical disorders have been selected for brief discussion.

Cystic fibrosis Cystic fibrosis is a complex disorder affecting various bodily systems, but particularly the lungs, where it causes recurrent infection and progressive damage, and to a lesser extent the pancreas, leading to difficulties in digesting and absorbing food. It may present soon after birth with meconium ileus (intestinal obstruction due to abnormal consistency of the gut contents at birth) or later with recurrent chest infections and failure to thrive. The most serious problem, the disease of the lungs, usually led in the past to death in childhood.

Although cystic fibrosis is the commonest serious inherited disease of childhood, its underlying cause is still not fully understood. Recent research suggests that the problem relates to the way in which chloride ions, necessary elements for many biological functions, are handled by secretory cells; and has located the cystic fibrosis gene on chromosome 7, bringing accurate antenatal diagnosis much nearer.

A recent BPA Report on Cystic Fibrosis (1986) gives an accurate picture of how the disease affects children in the UK. It occurs in about one child in 2000, and there are about 230 children born each year with the condition. About 80 per cent of these live till age ten, and about half reach adult life. Good liaison is therefore needed between the child and adult services to ensure continuity of care for these young adults.

The treatment which has improved the outlook in cystic fibrosis is care of the chest, with physiotherapy, vigorous antibiotic treatment of infections, and the maintenance of nutrition with enzyme supplements to replace the enzyme the pancreas is not producing, combined with a high-calorie diet. Current discussions about cystic fibrosis concern the best ways to use antibiotics and special diets or alternative feeding methods, and the value of neonatal screening. There is now a practicable method for such screening but the benefits of very early detection are not universally agreed. As in other disorders where the average paediatrician will only have a small number of cases under his care the question arises as to whether children with cystic fibrosis are best looked after in specialist centres. The BPA Report has suggested a compromise arrangement whereby local paediatricians cooperate with such centres so that geographical convenience is combined with the advantages of more specialized care in deciding what is best for a particular child.

Diabetes Diabetes mellitus affects rather more than one child per 1000, and is probably becoming commoner, particularly in socially advantaged children. Childhood diabetes is almost invariably 'insulin dependent'. The cause is probably a combination of a genetic predisposition and a precipitating factor in the environment, probably viral infection but possibly dietary.

The care of the diabetic child involves two priorities which, without skill and cooperation on the part of parents, child, and doctors, may conflict with each other. The first relates to the fact that diabetes is a lifelong disease. When it starts in childhood, the span of life available for developing the serious long-term complications affecting the eyes, kidneys, and arterial circulation is long. There are therefore very strong reasons for doing everything possible to prevent these disabling complications. This means strict diabetic control—care over the diet, administration of insulin in a way that will keep blood sugar levels as normal as possible (by injections more than once daily or by use of a continuous infusion pump), and frequent measurement of blood rather then urine glucose levels. Treatment is demanding on the child and family. The second consideration is to keep the child happy, emotionally stable, and with a social and school life not too disrupted by the demands of the disease and its treatment. In the past (when the treatment was often less intensive), diabetic children were sometimes disturbed in early childhood and rebellious in adolescence. The biochemical and psychosocial parts of management are both important and cannot be separated.

Impact of chronic handicap on the individual and the family

How handicap becomes apparent

There are three ways in which handicap can impinge upon a family, determined by the manner and timing of the realization that the child has an infirmity that will not go away.

The baby who is different from birth   The birth of an obviously abnormal child creates an immediate crisis, most acutely for the parents, but also affecting the wider family group and close neighbours. Doctors and nurses present at such a birth, however experienced, are invariably emotionally involved to some extent and their own, often deep and unacknowledged feelings will influence the way they act and speak.

An unusual appearance immediately alerts parents to the inevitability of a life of diminished potential and the possibility of multiple problems that can affect the lives of the whole family.

Down's syndrome is the most common condition producing this early confrontation with abnormality and handicap. In most cases, the condition is recognized at a glance by someone present in the delivery suite. Mothers describe vividly how their first inkling that something was amiss was an unusual staff grouping in the labour ward. Instead of the baby being wrapped up and handed to mother immediately after mouth secretions had been sucked out, and the midwives attending to other duties, a hushed group congregates round the cot in the corner while the mother is left by herself experiencing increasing anxiety.

Much attention has been paid in the last ten to fifteen years to the painful problems surrounding such an event. It is now realized that efforts to protect the feelings of the vulnerable new mother can, in fact, cause her confusion and sometimes resentment, and be seen as indifference or deception. The realization that a child has a disorder as indelible as Down's syndrome will provoke grief in most ordinary parents. Such grief is in no way abnormal. It is sometimes preceded by a stunned silence or later perhaps expressed as anger towards others, particularly a doctor thought responsible. The mother may react towards the child with fear or treat him as something alien. One mother said her baby was like a 'child from Mars', the modern equivalent to the myth of the changeling child left by the fairies when they stole the real one. There is no evidence that a grief reaction as such will precipitate a puerperal psychosis (psychiatric disturbance, usually temporary, after birth), a condition that still produces serious anxiety in the staff of obstetric departments. Severe post-partum psychiatric illness is not more common in those who have given birth to an abnormal child, and minor and more chronic depressive reactions are encountered only slightly more frequently than in mothers coping with normal babies in untoward environmental conditions such as poor housing and lack of warm supportive relationships.

There is no perfect, or foolproof, way to deal with very distressed human beings under any circumstances, but a number of recent studies of parental reactions have suggested some guidelines (Cunningham, Morgan, and McGucken 1984) for handling the breaking of such bad news. The problem differs in certain important respects from dealing with a death because of the continued presence of the child and the long-term responsibility facing the parents and likely to call for great personal resources. The guidelines for a 'model service' suggest first that as soon as possible the news of the handicap should be broken to the parents together in privacy by the consultant paediatrician, preferably with an appropriate member of the hospital nursing staff and a health visitor present. The baby should be in the room. Information should be given directly and plenty of time allowed for questions. This initial interview should be followed up by another the following day, after the parents have had time to digest the news and talk together in private. The mother's health visitor will go on seeing the family for practical advice and support, with a telephone number provided for emergencies.

Down's syndrome, in many cases, differs from other crises that occur early in an infant's life, because of the long-term implications accompanied by the lack of opportunity for immediate action and resulting helplessness.

Other conditions, apparent at birth, call for immediate and heroic surgery. Under these circumstances, despite the acute periods of worry, most parents cope well at the time, being comforted by the feeling that something is being done. The parents, however, may have to be away from home a lot and their other children may miss them and have difficulty empathizing with the anxiety their parents feel for someone they themselves do not yet know. Small siblings of sick or handicapped babies are not immune from feelings of rejection and jealousy. Parents may feel torn between their needs and concern for the new sick child. Resentment born then can persist, marring family relationships for years.

For babies with spina bifida, early dramatic action, comforting at the time, may be followed by the realization that the price paid by the children themselves does not always justify the early optimism.

A combination of an obvious abnormality with a prognosis of lasting handicap with another disorder lethal unless treated by immediate surgery produces the most difficult ethical dilemmas. Once more, Down's syndrome is the condition in which this situation most commonly arises, because of the high incidence of other abnormalities, such as atresia of the gut (localized absence of patency leading to obstruction) for which decisions regarding surgery have to be made.

The gradual recognition of handicap   The second type of confrontation with handicap for parents is when a child looks normal, is initially welcomed as such, but later shows evidence that there is something seriously amiss. The timing can vary enormously. At one extreme is an overlap with the previous group where a father, not having seen the baby, rushes to the telephone to announce the good news and then, elation having been replaced by depression, has to cope with the fact of abnormality and suffer the pain of disenchanting all those with whom he had earlier rejoiced.

More frequent are those cases in which a baby is nursed in the Special Care Baby Unit where, initially, hope is high that, like others apparently similar, he will grow up normally after a somewhat inauspicious start. As time goes on, with recovery slowing up, disquieting events occur, such as fits, or a never-ending sequence of complications, and hope gradually dwindles. There is no one moment, or even day, on which the parents realize that brain damage is present. The violent impact described above does not occur and the shock and grief can remain unacknowledged and unresolved. Even so, looking back some years later, most parents of children with demonstrable brain damage following birth injury feel they had come to terms with the fact that there had been permanent damage by the time the baby was a few months old.

Mental retardation, without obvious physical signs or stigmata, is much more difficult to recognize. The first visit of the mother anxiously seeking reassurance about her baby's normality will have been preceded by much private anguish and frantic comparison with the progress of other people's babies. Failure to develop speech and, in particular, a sense of being unable to 'get through' to the child are even more worrying to parents than delay in reaching motor 'milestones' of development. It is often difficult for the parents to pin-point when they thought something was definitely wrong. They are likely to meet reassurance at first from the primary care team (general practitioner, clinic doctor, health visitor, district nurse) who are afraid to label a child wrongly as backward. Well-meant comforting remarks often make a mother feel she is dismissed as fussy and can lead to a reluctance to return. It is common to hear such a mother say later that she had known something was wrong and yet nobody believed her, even though her doctor had taken the problem seriously from the start.

The next stage, when parents and primary care team agree that the child is significantly different from others, is the search for a diagnosis. Before a definite answer can be found, parents frequently experience a 'prediagnostic' anxiety. Any article in a paper or any television programme on disorders in children adds fuel to their burning need to find if there is something that can be removed or added to make it all better. For almost half of the children with mental retardation, no clear-cut answer will be found. Some parents gradually come to terms with the fact that there is no medical explanation and accept that the child is just generally backward, whilst others will continue for many years to search for the elusive diagnostic label.

The child who is firmly placed in the family before the fact of his or her retardation is recognized is unlikely to be regarded as a stranger or changeling, as sometimes is the new-born with an obvious abnormal appearance. The reaction of society is similar to that of parents. Children, normal in appearance but with quite severe retardation, will be accepted into playgroups and given the opportunity to start in mainstream education, while children of comparable ability but with obvious stigmata, for example of Down's syndrome, will not. However, acceptance into society is not invariably in the interest of the child and his family. Mothers of retarded children with normal appearance may report highly critical comments from strangers when the child misbehaves in public in contrast to the tolerance or special treatment—such as being rushed through the supermarket check-out—that is often offered to the more obviously handicapped child.

The absence of a diagnosis may lead to parental frustration and a sense of being to blame for failure to thrive or slow milestones. A diagnostic 'label', even one carrying a poor prognosis, can lead to parents feeling that they have been in some way exonerated.

The acquisition of a diagnostic label usually ends the search. The diagnosis can open the door to a parents' self-help organization, an important source of support and information.

Catastrophe hitting a previously normal child   A third and dramatic way in which handicap can strike a family is when a child who is normal for a few years suffers some catastrophe, such as sudden illness or trauma which destroys 'normality', leaving a damaged child. Head injury at birth has already been referred to as a possible cause of mental handicap and cerebral palsy. Severe head injuries, usually from road traffic accidents, are also an important cause of mental and/or physical disablement, which is often permanent in older children and adolescents.

Initially, after severe head trauma there is much action. The wonders of modern neurosurgery sustain early hope. The gradual let-down as hope fades and the parents find themselves going from high technological glamour to the opposite end of the spectrum, the inability of medicine to prevent sequelae, the paucity of facilities medical and other for the young chronic sick, is often painful. The grief that had been held in check during the very anxious period of the acute illness can be intense when there appears to be little more to do and, as in the case of the new-born, may well be directed outwards finding its expression as hostility towards anyone who may be considered to have caused the damage to the child or failed to provide a remedy. The problem of litigation is intertwined with understandable grief following catastrophes of this sort.

Grief is particularly liable to reach morbid intensity following a difficult or ambivalent relationship with a child prior to the disaster.

Occasionally the family may believe the child will die and go through a process of anticipatory grieving before death. When death does not occur and the survivor is almost unrecognizable as the loved and mourned child, the parents may have great difficulty establishing a new relationship. In some cases, one parent can succeed in this difficult task of adjustment and the other cannot, leading to immense strain in the marital relationship. The situation is often experienced in two extreme ways, as binding a couple very closely or driving a wedge between them.

Both child and parents can feel intensely cheated when a lasting handicap develops after what had been thought to be curative treatment for a life-threatening disorder. Children have been 'cured' of leukaemia, but then been found to be mentally retarded. Life-saving drugs for severe infections may produce profound deafness, resented bitterly by the sufferer, while the original disorder which the drug cured is forgotten.

Demands put upon parents

Handicap may impose perpetual childhood, first experienced as the long years in nappies of those slow to acquire continence, spoon-feeding at every meal, lifting when the weight becomes great, and no let-up in the need to supervise. All this has been carefully documented in recent research which indicates that, despite many improvements in other provision for many varieties of handicap, the bulk of sheer hard work remains within the family, in most cases falling on the mother.

Fear of the future and the prospect of a handicapped child never achieving independence and never being able to leave home haunt older parents. The cost of alternative permanent shelter, such as village communities or home farm trusts, is prohibitive and the length of the waiting list is long. Local social service departments which may be trying to set up local facilities can appear to be unfeeling if they refuse to support the chosen private scheme. Plans have to be made in advance and even parents who have worked hard for years to raise funds to meet the cost of a particular facility, such as a community for autistic children, may find that when their time comes their own child is not considered suitable.

Early intervention, involving specialized teaching of the child in the home in the pre-school years, is now practiced in many countries, using a variety of models and methods. Most common in this country is the Portage method, in which a trained home teacher visits the home and instructs the mother how to teach her child in carefully defined steps. There is no doubt that such early intervention is beneficial, not just to the child but also to the parents. Being treated as partners in the education and therapy of their handicapped child is a vast improvement on being left helpless with an 'untreatable' child. Some parents, however, usually because of many other problems besetting them, are unable to cope with the demands of an early intervention programme such as Portage. Other, less formal methods may be more successful. A very different sort of parent, used to solving life's problems, can react sharply to what is seen as either patronizing or intrusive in the regular visits of the home teacher. At each Child Development Centre a flexible approach to early intervention needs to be adopted with Portage as one useful option.

Other forms of therapy, such as speech therapy or physiotherapy, now often require parents to learn the exercises and practice them with the child. The increased chance of success if fulfilled is very rewarding, but such parental involvement requires motivation and an ability to understand what is required.

In the treatment of severe behaviour disorders, secondary to handicap, success will be short-lived without the full participation of parents. In the past, children have been admitted to units, treated intensively, and their distressing behaviour modified, only to relapse on returning home to the profound disappointment and humiliation of the parents who are then even less able to cope than before. To combat this, parents are now closely involved in planning the intervention, must if necessary keep in close touch throughout the admission, and then take the major responsibility for keeping the prescribed treatment going.

Treatment of a handicapped child demands great commitment from parents. Some parents find such commitment worthwhile and are convinced of the efficacy of treatment which may make great demands on them, despite lack of objective scientific evidence that the treatment itself is better than other less demanding forms or even no treatment at all. Belief that the treatment will work is an important factor determining the outcome.

Although most parents greatly welcome this active participation, there is a limit to the endurance of them all. They must be able to see what their work can lead to and they must have the chance of time off with effective relaxation. Physically disabled or retarded children who are born into families with many existing problems are at a particular disadvantage.

Involvement of parents in management of services for handicapped children

Many of the improvements in services for the handicapped of all ages are due to the activities of parents and the increasing recognition that their voice should be heard by administrators and politicians. Parent representation on committees of management, such as of Portage teams, special schools, and local authority hostels, ensures that the provision of services is relevant and of a high standard.

The active participation of parents in the running of respite services has been found to be successful. It is sometimes feared that the more vociferous families will take over the service, to the detriment of other more needy but more reticent parents. Yet, it is found that the more demanding are more likely to modify their requests when the need for fair shares is put to them by other parents rather than by professionals. The other advantage of strong parent participation is that inter-service squabbles, such as between local authority departments of Education and Social Services can be minimized.

In the management of handicap it is essential to take the individual characteristics of the child and family into consideration, since needs vary widely. Some families have remarkably little need of outside services, managing their handicapped child as part of the self-contained family. Yet even the most self-sufficient can need an advocate. Parents who are too self-sufficient can find that their independence is a disadvantage. There can still be an attitude where services are provided in the form of a *table d'hote* menu, that parents are expected to take all the package of services for the handicapped or receive none. This is neither good care nor good economics.

A more active and questioning attitude of parents is seen too in the medical sphere. In some instances, (e.g. correction of facial stigmata by plastic surgery) parents are showing a tendency to prefer the advice of a parent support group rather than medical opinion.

Foster and adoptive parents also need services, including the opportunity of respite services. Mixing natural parents and foster or adoptive parents in discussion groups can pose problems, but the energy of the volunteer group who have chosen to take on the care of handicapped children is useful in parent/teacher associations and in improving services.

Alternative parenting

The parenting of a child with a severe and lasting disability is a lifelong task, with which not everyone can cope. The future can seem utterly hopeless, particularly to those confronted with a handicap before they have had time to get to know the child with it. How many cannot begin to cope? The estimates, of 10 to 12 per cent, are remarkably similar from area to area and do not seem to be influenced to a great degree by the quality of the early services available. Occasionally there appears in one geographical area to be an excess of parents who do not wish to take their child home to be part of their family. Little is known of the factors leading to such an action, since the parents rarely agree to being interviewed after the event and before it the anxiety of all around is such that a questioning outsider is thought likely to jeopardize the situation still further. Psychiatrists, even those with special expertise in families with handicapped children, are often excluded deliberately. This would seem to be an uninformed attitude.

In recent years *adoption* of handicapped children has become a real alternative to upbringing within the natural family. The evidence on rearing in institutions is such that it is no longer ethical to admit a small child to a long-stay hospital. A clash of interests can then arise, since it is sometimes very difficult for mothers to accept placement in someone else's home. The feeling they experience is 'If I can't mother him, he must be unmotherable'. Admission to a hospital supports the view that the child needs special care of a type which no family can provide or that such a child is so handicapped that he has no appreciation and hence no need of the loving ties with members of a family. Seeing the handicapped child thrive in the care of a foster mother, and respond to her love, can be extremely painful for the biological mother. None the less, the child's needs must take priority, although the pain of the natural parents must be appreciated, and sometimes treated.

Many adoption agencies find little difficulty in placing small babies with Down's syndrome for adoption. There are many couples longing for a child, and the dearth of normal babies available for adoption has meant that the small child with a recognized disability now has a very good chance of finding a permanent home. The parents, of course, are volunteers and do not experience the grief that giving birth to a defective child brings. They are usually well informed before they take the baby and then well-supported by social workers or, better still, by other adoptive parents who have made the same sort of decision. The people who take this step are often strong characters with very definite views. Some have had previous experience of similar handicap. The results are very good, with the children doing at least as well as those brought up in their own family homes, and markedly better than those brought up in any sort of institution.

Following the success of adoption of small babies with an obvious disability, older children with handicaps are now being placed for adoption usually by specialist agencies. The older handicapped child may need a new family because of the breakdown of the family of birth, an event now so common that it cannot so often be attributed justifiably to the presence of the handicapped child. Unfortunately the child is an obvious scapegoat, if not by the parents then by others with outmoded ideas. Thus an older handicapped child is more likely to have had traumatic personal experience and be doubly handicapped by the presence of emotional or behavioural disorder. There are, however, people who are willing to foster, and even adopt, such difficult and, at first sight, unrewarding children. The substitute parents who volunteer for and succeed in this task often possess qualities derived from overcoming personal hardship. They are rarely the sort of parents that immediately spring to mind as ideal adoptive parents. Many single people have succeeded in this task as have older couples who have already brought up their own families.

Fostering lacks the permanent commitment of adoption, but there are various types of fostering that are very useful in the care of handicapped children. In many areas there is now a hospitality scheme in which a host family is chosen to match the family of the handicapped child. Instead of respite care in a hostel or hospital, the child goes as a welcome visitor to a family he or she knows well, similar to visiting a loved relative. The scheme can be flexible to include brothers and sisters and often a warm friendship develops between the two families. However, matching need not be too close since many children gain from contrasting experience, such as going to a happy-go-lucky household with lots of children from one with many other advantages but less company and perhaps less acceptance. Another example of the use of fostering is shared care, which can sometimes develop from a hospitality arrangement. Here a child who is particularly difficult spends a larger proportion of his time with the host family, but retains important links with home. This arrangement is also useful where there is a single parent, a particularly impoverished or unstimulating home, or where parental or sibling interests can be conflicting.

Brothers and sisters of handicapped children

There is little evidence from recent research that the presence of a handicapped child in a family has an inevitable detrimental effect on the other children. The improvement in attitudes and services has lifted some of the relentless 'burden of care' described 20 or more years ago. Parents who are fond and resourceful with regard to their normal children are likely to show the same attributes to their handicapped children, and vice versa. Rarely is one excessively indulged and the other relatively neglected. More often a lack of parental skills will be evident in the rearing of normal as well as handicapped, but it is usually the child with disability who will be the most vulnerable.

The relationships between family factors, such as health of the parents, environmental factors such as poverty and poor housing, and behavioural and emotional reactions in handicapped children and their normal siblings, are complex. The notion of 'stress' in families producing disorder in other members is over-simplistic. Handicap in some families can produce strengths hitherto dormant. In others, particularly those with weak marital relationships, what superficially looks like a similar degree of handicap can be very destructive.

Several further points are important. An accumulation of adverse factors such as poverty, poor housing, and lack of a stable and confiding relationship compounded by a handicapped child have an effect that is more than the sum of the individual factors, the strain on the family members increasing exponentially. Certain types of mental retardation usually said to be the milder types are more common in more disadvantaged families, but these children may function at a level comparable to children with more severe, clearly defined syndromes from more stimulating and less stressed homes. Milder degrees of similar problems, such as learning difficulties, will be common in the siblings from such disadvantaged families, adding to the vulnerability of the family as a whole.

Problems of emotion and behaviour in handicapped children

Handicapped children, like their normal brothers and sisters, react to family influences. An emotional reaction to a stress may be expressed in an unusual way. For example, grief following loss due to bereavement or parental separation may take the form of aggression, sometimes directed towards the remaining parent. The concept of death is too difficult to grasp, but the loss is still felt acutely. Disturbance in the retarded child may then cause a reaction in a brother or sister, or discord between parents, thus producing effects in both directions. Treatment of the reactive behavioural disorder in isolation from the rest of the family is unlikely to be successful.

The repertoire of behaviours in retarded children is wider than that found commonly in children in the normal intellectual range. They can show bizarre mannerisms, regression, or even apparent psychotic behaviour, as well as the tears, tantrums, and quarrels seen in their siblings. Symptoms often last longer with children still angry or clinging months after mother's brief absence. On other occasions, such as when all the rest of the family are upset by an event, the handicapped child fails to see it as disturbing, carrying on as before.

Behaviour problems of significant severity to upset most ordinary families are common, occurring in one-third to one-half of retarded children. They are more common in the more severely handicapped, are particularly associated with inability to communicate, and show only minor variations in incidence between diagnoses.

All children with peculiarities, chronic disorders, or disabilities have an increased risk of behavioural and emotional problems, but the risk of psychiatric disorder is particularly high in those disorders with actual malformation or damage above the brain stem.

Adolescence

Because of the increased dependence during childhood and concern over the degree of independence possible in adulthood, passage into adult life is fraught with anxiety for handicapped children. Parents commonly find it difficult to accept the maturation of a dependent child, denying emerging sexuality and failing to face up to consideration of a life away from them. These difficulties are much increased by the poor services available after school, both for physically handicapped and mentally retarded youngsters. The children's services experienced during the school years are seen in retrospect as a protection that falls away to nothing, although extension of education to the age of 19 years is an important provision.

It is essential to talk to the handicapped adolescent explaining the disability. As a child, he has probably been used to being talked about, but has rarely had his problems discussed directly with him. Emotional subjects and embarrassing issues may have to be discussed in privacy without fear of disclosure and away from an ever-present mother. Adolescent needs may have been overlooked while the family coped with the various manifestations of the disability. Parents who have been devoted carers can be deeply hurt and very angry when they are first confronted by the adolescent's understandable need to be rid of them occasionally.

These problems are often tackled in an imaginative way in the 'leavers' class' in special schools. However, handicapped children in mainstream education can be overlooked where there are larger numbers and much is taken for granted. Medical services continuing the care of the adolescent must understand their needs. At present there is little interaction between the various departments caring for the medical needs of adults with handicap, and adolescents tend to be merely tossed into these. The medical care of the adolescent with long-term disability is unsatisfactory and needs radical improvement.

Care of handicapped children and their families

Needs of handicapped children and their families

The handicapped child makes different demands on a health service from the child with an acute illness. The family of a handicapped child becomes intimately involved with the process of their child's chronic problem and this clearly also has implications for the health services. In this section we shall first review the needs of the handicapped and then consider how health and other services meet these needs.

The needs are:
1. Early identification of the impairment.
2. Diagnosis.
3. Assessment (noting the strengths as well as the weaknesses of the child and the family).

4. Immediate practical advice. Counselling of the handicapped person/family.
5. Programme for the management of the child: (a) management of the handicap, (b) treatment of the treatable.
6. 'Normal child rearing'.
7. Periodic reassessment.

Early identification of handicap   In many instances a congenital disorder will be recognized by the parent(s) and their attendants at birth (e.g. spina bifida). Sometimes the attendants may realize that something is wrong when the parents do not. The classic example of this is Down's syndrome where the facies are distinctive enough for the experienced professional to identify the disorder but often not abnormal enough to alert the parents. In other situations a routine test may identify the problem (e.g. certain metabolic disorders).

Sometimes a child will appear normal at birth, but abnormal or delayed development will eventually lead the parent to guess that all is not well. There are those who feel that where a handicapping condition is untreatable early identification is not helpful either to parents or child. Some doctors in the past delayed telling parents that their child had Down's syndrome until the parents became worried about the child's development. We believe that is policy is almost invariably wrong. Hippocrates first suggested that it was the doctor's job to understand the nature of the disease and know its course. The doctor's ability to identify *correctly* that something is wrong and to tell the patient or his family about the possible consequences raises the confidence in the doctor and allows him to be a more effective counsellor and friend to child and family. Further, early diagnosis may lead to effective treatment or amelioration of some potentially handicapping illnesses and/or secondary problems (such as contractures in cerebral palsy and secondary emotional disturbance in the family). The closer in time diagnosis is to the insult causing damage the better is the understanding of causation likely to be. A service needs to provide the earliest possible identification of handicap.

Diagnosis   Diagnosis involves clinical examination of the child together with such relevant investigations as required. Investigations may take many forms.

In the past doctors often too readily accepted many cases of mental retardation as inexplicable, but if fully investigated at least a partial explanation of the cause can be achieved in many cases. Parents want to know the cause of their child's problem providing the child is not submitted to unpleasant procedures. Now that there are effective non-invasive methods of investigating children every effort should be made to identify the cause of handicapping conditions. Such investigations, apart from providing specific information for the family, may also lead to more understanding of the condition and potentially its prevention.

Diagnostic procedures should not be repeated heedlessly and should not be allowed to drag on over months or even years. A diagnosis may, however, need review, and new techniques may develop which make further investigation desirable. With 'late' diagnostic procedures parents (rightly) often take a lot of persuading that these are going to prove helpful to the child.

Diagnostic procedures usually require the facilities of a hospital.

Assessment Diagnosis looks to the cause(s) of a condition but does not necessarily give a picture of the child's functioning. A child with Down's syndrome may have near normal intellectual functioning or be profoundly retarded. In planning a programme for a handicapped child a knowledge of his/her level of functioning is essential. Assessment is age-related and needs to be repeated periodically. It is customary to review the child's function in different aspects; i.e. gross and fine motor function, vision, hearing, speech, language, perceptual/intellectual, social/emotional.

The problem of assessing a child will depend on his disorder. The motor function of a child with cerebral palsy may be difficult to assess, while his vision *may* be normal and easy to assess.

Assessment requires staff with special skills at assessing particular functions (e.g. a physiotherapist to assess motor function) but at the same time it is important to obtain a good overall picture of the child.

Immediate practical advice/counselling Parents confronted with a handicapped child need information about the nature of the child's condition and counsel/comfort as they cope with their own stress and grief about the child's condition. They also want at once to be involved in helping their child and advised as to what they can do. As the handicapped child grows he/she also needs to be able to talk to and discuss with an informed counsellor about his/her feelings and frustrations.

Telling parents about a diagnosis implying handicap is often badly done. Experience and training are needed if the continuing task of counselling is to be done sensitively.

Children, handicapped or normal, have different needs at different ages. In the early years these include the achievement of normal daily living skills such as feeding and continence skills. The child develops mobility at these early ages. Language, of course, is another major achievement of the pre-school years. Academic skills like reading are acquired later. A programme to help a child achieve maximal potential should be based on the normal child's development but progress may be much slower. Achieving goals is important, with regular revision of aims.

Management   The aim of management of handicap is to ameliorate as far as possible and to prevent secondary problems. Thus the cerebral palsied child may develop dislocated hips if not positioned and handled appropriately. Where the child cannot achieve independent mobility (i.e. is wheel-chair bound) the most effective chair must be provided. The needs of the child clearly change as he gets older. The most important need at school age may be appropriate management of a learning disorder, while later measures to enable the handicapped to achieve open employment, if possible, may be most necessary.

Treatment of the 'treatable'   By definition a handicap is chronic. Nevertheless a child with handicap may have symptoms which can be treated. Epilepsy, urinary tract infection in association with spina bifida, and visual acuity defects can often be treated successfully. Many handicapped people have additional treatable conditions. Visual and hearing conditions are often missed in handicapped populations.

Help with normal child rearing   All parents have some problems in rearing their young. Many parents of young babies, for example, have difficulties with feeding or there may be difficulties with sleep. Temper tantrums and other management problems are common as the child gets older. Schooling leads many parents to have anxieties about the educational progress of their child. The process of rearing a child involves a complex integration between the family—parents and child—and health, education, and social services. In developed countries with small nuclear families the state has taken to providing help for families.

The handicapped child has, of course, the same needs as a normal child, but his difficulties are often exacerbated. The family should have access to the normal forms of support as well as the special support that may be needed because of the handicap. The handicapped child may attend the local child health clinic and some of the problems may be dealt with there. Hopefully he will go to an ordinary school and the parents meet with the teachers as would ordinary parents. Parents of handicapped children often find it hard to believe that there are difficulties in rearing normal children and tend to believe that all their problems are linked to their child's handicap.

Periodic reassessment   While diagnosis and diagnostic procedures can be completed initially it is very often impossible to predict how the handicapped child will develop functionally. At periodic intervals reassessment is necessary. The timing of this may vary from child to child but there are certain obvious and appropriate times—in the four-to-five years age group before entering formal education, at the age of nine or ten before puberty and the move to a secondary school, and at thirteen or fourteen years for an assessment of post-school needs.

There is also need to reassess the child on other occasions. If orthopaedic surgery has been undertaken (which hopefully might mean a major change in the child's mobility activities) it would be sensible six months later to reassess the child's motor functions. This might involve replanning some other aspects of life. The need for physiotherapy may have diminished and more help be required for other aspects of development.

Reassessment may involve not only the child but the situation of the whole family. The birth of further children, changes in parental occupation, health problems of other members of the family, and marital problems may also have to be considered. All these will have implications for the development of the handicapped child and make it appropriate to undertake reassessment at a particular time rather than at the times suggested above.

How the needs are met

Where should the child be seen?
A decision needs to be taken on where a handicapped child should be seen—home, hospital, school—who are going to be involved, and what services are offered. It is worth having some regard to the role of those who work with handicapped children and the amount of time that they spend with them. Doctors and other professionals such as psychologists tend to see the child relatively rarely (perhaps once every three months or so), but often initiate major changes in the child's circumstances, recommending, for example, that they should go to a special school or have a surgical operation. As these professionals are usually highly trained, few in number, and expensive, they spend relatively little time with the handicapped child. Another group of people, parents, houseparents, teachers, and therapists, may work with a child over long periods of time and have repeated contact with him yet play little part in altering the circumstances of the child's life. The different groups of professionals must meet together and see that they are in accord about decisions made. From early on too it is important to see that the child, as well as the parents, is part of the decision-making process. It is not easy for teachers to attend a case conference at a hospital, but with a school-aged child decisions made without the participation of staff actually involved are probably rather pointless. Whereas in the pre-school period therefore it is reasonable to examine the child in health facilities, in the school period the team needs to be part of the school the child attends. While the personnel in the Child Development Centre may not be able to attend regularly all school-based meetings, they should ensure that representatives of the District Handicap Team do so.

Another issue arising commonly with the handicapped child is the reliability of observations of function at a clinic visit and the parents' description of the child's functioning at home. In many instances a thorough picture of the child's functional ability is best obtained by observing the child in the home situation. The home is the parents' 'ground' where they feel at ease, where the doctor is an intruder. He may feel uneasy there. It is easier for parents to relate to people they have met at home and, although it is difficult to make regular home visits, in our view time spent doing this, at least once, pays enormous dividends in the developing relationship between the family and its medical advisors.

Health facilities

Paediatrics as a specialty only became established in this country in the 1930s and 1940s and even then the number of paediatricians was small. Children with handicaps were seen in ordinary out-patient departments. Over the years it has come to be realized that a half-hour appointment in a busy out-patient department is hardly appropriate for the full diagnostic and functional assessment of the child. The Court Report (1976) recommended that special arrangements should be made for the care of handicapped children. It proposed the setting up of District Handicap Teams which would include not only paediatricians and nurses but also physiotherapists, speech and occupational therapists, a psychologist, and teachers. It was suggested that the District Handicap Teams should relate to the Regional Centre. Over the years since the Court Report two thirds of the districts in England and Wales have developed District Handicap Teams. Backing these District Handicap Teams the Court Report recognized the need for the Regional Centres where more complex diagnostic procedures would be available and where the staff would have additional skills. Most Regional Centres, for example, would expect to have a paediatric neurologist on their staff.

Services for the identification of handicap   While many handicaps can be identified in the neonatal period many cannot. To ensure that potentially handicapping conditions are not missed every baby should be examined by a paediatrically trained doctor in the neonatal period. Thereafter children will be assessed in the community. In recent years Child Health Clinics, often run by District Health Authorities and staffed by doctors and health visitors they employ, have played a major part in the surveillance of the population with a view to identifying handicap early. In the future many of these clinics will probably be part of general practice, although in the large urban areas, with inadequate general practice cover and many unregistered young parents, health authority clinics with an appropriate geographical distribution will probably need to persist. A very important person within these services is the health visitor, who may be responsible for much of the surveillance work. The ages at which children should be regularly surveyed has been the subject of much debate but most people favour around six weeks, six to eight months, at least once towards the end of the second year of life, at three years, and on entry to school at age five.

Given more widely disseminated knowledge of normal child development the best people to survey a child's development are probably the parents. They need easy access to trained doctors and nurses so that as soon as any parental anxiety is present it can be evaluated by a trained professional. Professional staff should be competent to assess a child at any age and tell the parents whether or not they think the development is normal. There are, however, limitations. Early predictors of language delay, for example, are unreliable: the development of language cannot be assessed adequately until the time at which it should be present. Similarly although there are some predictors of learning disorders these are by no means reliable and regular periodic review of children is essential if problems of this nature are going to be identified as they arise. Commonly referrals of children with such problems are much too late so that reading delays reach psychologists and doctors for advice when the child is nine, ten, or eleven years, by which time a sense of failure has been built into the child's life. Easy access, by teachers, to developmental paediatricians and psychologists in the early years of education would mean that as soon as a child had difficulties in a learning process skilled help could be brought to his aid.

Many minor developmental delays will be seen in Child Health and General Practitioner Clinics in the pre-school years and by no means all of them need be referred to a District Handicap Team. Between 10 and 15 per cent of children have evident speech and language delay at three years (not talking in sentences and having a restricted vocabulary). Some of these children are merely at the lower end of the range of normality. In others there is a reason for their delayed development such as, for example, the presence of otitis media (infection of the ear affecting hearing). The majority of these children will be helped by the local Child Health Clinic. Only the 1 or 2 per cent of children with more severe handicaps will be referred on to the District Handicap Team.

The district handicap team While there are arguments for siting District Handicap Teams on educational sites there are strong reasons for concluding that the best site is within the ambit of a District General Hospital. Not only are diagnostic facilities readily at hand but it is also easier then to obtain the services of relevant consultants such as orthopaedic surgeons and ophthalmologists. Children may be referred direct to the District Handicap Team from the neonatal nursery or referred from Child Health Clinics and family doctors for assessment and management. The types of disorder which are commonly seen by District Handicap Teams are set out in Table 4.1.

Table 4.1

Diagnosis commonly seen by child development centres. The diagnoses are listed in order of frequency. Some centres also see children with cystic fibrosis, asthma, and congenital heart disease, which may or may not be appropriate. [Based on data collected by Bax and Whitemore, (1985).]

Diagnosis
Mentally handicapped (excluding Down's syndrome)
Learning disorders (excluding intellectually retarded)
Epilepsy
Children with behavioural problems
Language disorders
Cerebral palsy
Down's syndrome
Blind/partially sighted
Spina bifida
Deaf/partially hearing
Muscular dystrophy
Autistic /psychotic
Arthrogryposis (and many other equally uncommon diagnoses)

The essential difference between the operation of the District Handicap Team and the ordinary out-patient department is that in the former the child can be assessed by a range of disciplines. Ample time should be available for the parents to understand the processes that are going on and to take a full part with the team in assessing the child and in planning what help he needs and how it is to be obtained. Preferably the siting of the District Handicap Team should be within easy reach of the parents as travelling long distances with a handicapped child can be very difficult and, in addition, after initial assessment members of staff may wish to pay visits to the home to help develop appropriate management. Certainly physiotherapists and occupational therapists will want to do this, and usually the doctor as well.

The handicapped child has a statutory right to pre-school education from the age of two. A decision has to be made as to whether he/she can enter an ordinary pre-school provision, as many if not most are able to do, or whether he needs to have special provision. Special provision may be necessary for some time while needs are assessed and then hopefully transfer back to an ordinary nursery school will be possible.

The school-aged handicapped child The 1981 Education Act incorporated many of the recommendations of the Warnock Report (1978) which stressed the aim of integrated education for the handicapped child. By this it was meant that handicapped children should be educated in normal schools alongside healthy peers. This proposal caught the public's attention while the recognition within the Report that special schools would also need to continue was less regarded. Thus the aim of integration into ordinary schools has received great emphasis but whereas the integration of a handicapped child into an ordinary school virtually always requires additional staffing the 1981 Act is seldom implemented in respect of additional educational resources. The Act also states that handicapped children should only be integrated into ordinary schools if this can be done without adversely affecting normal children.

Another change of the 1981 Act was that it abolished categories of handicap such as visually handicapped, physically handicapped, deaf, maladjusted, and delicate and suggested that children should be described simply as having special educational needs. While the aim behind this was to see that children were broadly assessed and not simply slotted into categories, as tended to happen in the past, the result has been that it is now very difficult to get a clear picture of what the special needs are. A child who has been assessed does not appear on an educational programme with any diagnostic label attached to him and special schools no longer indicate the broad category of handicap with which they are concerned.

If more handicapped children are going to attend ordinary schools an appropriate health service must be available to meet their needs. Presently the School Health Service is under considerable reorganization and there is controversy about how it should develop. Every school requires a named doctor and nurse who provide the health cover in a school. The nurse will do much of the routine surveillance of school children involving regular testing of vision and hearing (the latter particularly in the young ages), watching children's height and weight, and generally advising the school when, for example, there are outbreaks of infections. All children should have a competent medical assessment around the age of five but after that the doctor's work will be seeing children who have difficulties, particularly of learning and behaviour, which affect their school performance and handicapped children to ensure that for them health care is integrated with educational plans. The School Health Service is part of the Community Paediatric Service but in ordinary schools the doctor might be a general practitioner with a special interest in child health or a doctor from the Community Paediatric Team. The problem with integration into ordinary schools is that children with complex problems such as spina bifida can be in ordinary schools staffed by a doctor without the necessary specialist training in all the complexities of the care of the spina bifida child. When children with moderate to severe handicaps were in special schools it was easy for a community paediatrician to be appointed as the school medical officer and plan to spend appropriate amounts of time there. With dispersal, providing an appropriate service is going to be more time-consuming and hence more expensive and this needs to be recognized.

The emphasis of health care for the school-aged handicapped child should move from the District Handicap Team and the hospital into the school so that those who spend most time with the handicapped child such as teachers and care staff are able to participate fully in the health professional's appraisals and recommendations about the child's care. Doctors who work in schools with handicapped children should also participate in the pre-school care of the handicapped child so that all the information collected by the District Handicap Team is available in the school. For individual children rereferral from time to time to the District Handicap Team in the hospital for specific tests or for specific treatment will be appropriate. Much health-oriented treatment such as physiotherapy and occupational and speech therapy should be provided for the child in school and integrated within his educational programme.

If teachers in ordinary schools are going to have moderately to severely handicapped children within their classrooms there are of course needs for additional educational resources which are recognized in the 1981 Act and all schools should have a teacher with training in special education available to advise and help with particular children. Schools nevertheless are also going to want access to health advice as to how to help particular children. While far more health training should be an essential part of the teacher training programmes the teacher is also going to learn on the job with the help of health professionals how to meet the needs of individual children; for example, how to deal with a partially hearing child. There is much work for health professionals to do within the classroom if handicapped children are going to get the services which they need.

Puberty, adolescence, and afterwards for the handicapped The handicapped child, like the non-handicapped, goes through all the normal processes of child rearing but puberty and adolescence may present particular difficulties. Achieving independence and satisfactory psychosexual adult life are not easy for the handicapped young person. Additional support is needed at this time. Prospects in adult life for an ordinary job and satisfactory wage-earning are precarious, particularly in a time of high unemployment. When the handicapped young persons eventually leave school, the school health service and much of the health support which they have had up to that time disappear. Many paediatricians and District Handicap Teams feel that they can no longer go on providing a service for them. Young mentally handicapped adults may be helped by Mental Handicap Teams which currently exist in the community but for the physically handicapped there is no such provision. We believe that all districts should have designated staff to look after young handicapped adults and see that they do not deteriorate, as many do at present, during late-adolescence and early adult life.

A flexible health service where staff with special knowledge of handicap are readily available seems an appropriate provision but this must be coupled with continuous contact as many of the handicapped young population may not themselves feel that they particularly want to make formal contact. They run the risk of getting lost to the health service. Informal relationships are important in detecting the early signs of deterioration.

Other organizations which help the handicapped   Both social service departments and educational services have statutory duties and service commitments to the handicapped, which we shall not detail here, but simply stress that there must be close cooperation between education, health, and social services.

In addition there are many agencies which may provide help for handicapped children. Of the quasi governmental agencies the most important is perhaps the Family Fund which the government finances but which is run through the Rowntree Trust. The Family Fund can provide financial help for families with handicapped children and this can range from additional medical aids to paying for a holiday or providing a family with an adaption to a car. The availability of such funds may be very significant in planning services for a handicapped child. Most handicaps now have a parent group associated with them, these groups ranging from very large and potentially powerful consumer organizations—like the Spastics Society which has an assessment centre where children may be seen by doctors and psychologists and a range of services such as special schools—to much smaller organizations where groups of parents with children with perhaps a rare disorder come together. Many of these parent groups know a great deal about the day-to-day problems of living with a handicapped child and they can pass this information on to other parents. Many such groups have a medical advisor who can be very helpful giving advice and information about particular problems.

Another major activity of voluntary organizations devoted to the handicapped has been to stimulate and fund *research*. With central funding for medical research becoming increasingly hard to obtain, the role of the medical charities has become more and more important. Often the establishment of research can be linked with some improvement in the service provided in a district, and, by setting the example of an excellent service with the help of some money from voluntary organizations, other districts may feel bound to follow this example and develop similar services from regular sources of income.

Voluntary organizations therefore can play a major role in 'pump priming' the ordinary services. In addition voluntary organizations can play an important part as pressure groups who regularly lobby to obtain improved funding of facilities for handicapped children. While there is increasing consumer participation in all aspects of the health service, perhaps nowhere has this been more prominent than with the handicapped. Parents have rightly felt that they have not been adequately helped. Paediatricians involved with the handicapped have to play their part in advocacy and in helping groups to formulate their needs clearly so that desired improvements in services can be achieved.

References

Bax, M. C. O. and Whitmore, K. (1985). District Handicap Teams: structure, functions and relationships. A report to the Department of Health and Social Service.

Court Report (1976). *Fit for the future. Report of the committee on Child Health Services.* Chairman: S. D. M. Court. HMSO, London.

Cunningham, C. C. Morgan, P. A. and McGucken, R. D. (1984) Down's syndrome: Is dissatisfaction with disclosure of diagnosis inevitable? *Developmental Medicine and Child Neurology* **26**, pp. 33-9.

Warnock Report (1978). *Special educational needs: report of the Committee of Enquiry into the Education of Handicapped Children and Young People.* Chairwomen: H. M. Warnock, Cmnd 7212, HMSO, London.

5

Child health and the environment

JEAN GOLDING, DAVID HULL,
and MICHAEL RUTTER

Introduction

Paediatrics is largely concerned with treating and curing illness in
children, but if disease is to be prevented and the health of the
childhood population improved it is important to understand the
factors associated with the genesis of disease. With the exception
of a few clear-cut disorders where there is a known direct causal
mechanism (bite by rabid animal and the development of rabies,
recessive genes and the development of cystic fibrosis), most
disorders are probably due to a combination of environmental
influences and genetic predisposition. In this chapter we are
concerned only with the identification of the most important facets
of the environment.

Physical environment

Geographic variation
The distribution of childhood illness varies from country to country.
Information on this is limited because ill health, whether physical
or psychological, is difficult to measure; without standard definitions
comparative data are meaningless. Information on hospital admissions exists, but this probably measures health-care facilities
and policy as much as morbidity.

Within Britain, national cohort studies have been able to collect
data on various disorders in children (Golding 1984). These studies
have followed nationally representative samples of births in 1946,
1958, and 1970 through childhood. An analysis of the first five
years of the latest cohort (Butler and Golding 1986) showed that
there were substantial variations in the types of illness between one
part of Britain and another. For example, in Wales children are
more likely to have upper and lower respiratory problems, repeated
headaches, and abdominal pains but less likely to report eczema

or hay fever. In Scotland, children are more likely to be admitted to hospital and twice as likely as the rest of the nation to have a tonsillectomy, but the reported prevalence of most disorders, such as abdominal pain, bronchitis, wheezing attacks, or headaches, is substantially lower than expected. Within England, once social conditions have been taken into account, there is no sign that living in the favoured south-east carries health benefits *per se*. Indeed the children from both the south-east and the south-west are significantly more likely to have hay fever.

Far greater differences are shown in the health behaviour of mothers. Mothers in Wales, Scotland and the northern parts of England are significantly less likely to breast-feed. Mothers in Scotland and the north and north-west regions of England are more likely to smoke, and to smoke heavily. Conversely Scottish children are more likely to have had the appropriate immunizations.

Such broad regional differences ignore the possible contrasts between urban and rural areas (Graham 1979). An early study (Rutter, Yule, Morton, and Bagley 1975) compared children living in an area of inner London with those on the mainly rural Isle of Wight. There were substantial differences in emotional and conduct disorders, apparently due to increased prevalence of parental mental disturbance, marital disruption, and discord in the inner city.

Cruder data from the 1970 national cohort study showed that parents living in inner urban areas were more likely to be immigrants, to move house frequently, to be single parents, heavy smokers, and of low social class. Although children living in such areas were significantly more likely to have a history of bed-wetting, temper tantrums, speech dysfluency (stammering/stuttering), repeated headaches, wheezing attacks, bronchitis, pneumonia, and habitual mouth breathing, almost all of these associations were considered to be related to the social characteristics of the residents. Nevertheless, residence in inner urban areas did appear to confer an independent increased risk of speech dysfluency, temper tantrums and habitual mouth breathing.

Climate

Long ago Hippocrates stated that children living in cities with a southern exposure were more likely to have asthma or epilepsy, whereas those in areas facing north were said to mature more slowly. Much of the variation he ascribed to the climate, the air breathed and the water drunk. These factors may still be important yet it is surprising how few studies have considered them.

Some causes of morbidity and death vary with the season of the year and hence are assumed to be associated with climatic conditions. The mechanisms are varied. Experimental studies show that house dust mites breed best when the temperature is about 25°C and the relative humidity about 80 per cent, in keeping with the observation that there is a high concentration of house dust mites during hot humid summers. This may well be a reason why the mortality rate from asthma peaks in August.

Many infectious diseases are more common in cold weather, including influenza and respiratory syncitial virus infection (a virus which particularly affects babies), but others such as para-influenza virus infection peak in the summer. The 'cause' of death with the greatest summer/winter differential is the sudden infant death syndrome (cot deaths). Whether observations are made in the northern or southern hemispheres the same pattern is found—the colder the time of year the higher the mortality. Nevertheless, within a given month deaths are not more likely to occur on the coldest days. A number of authors have attempted to find a pattern of climatic factors that might cluster together at the time of a sudden infant death, but so far to no avail.

An important question in any study of climate and morbidity concerns the natural human biochemical variation with season. One of the most striking is the variation associated with the lack of sunshine in the winter—resulting in reduced vitamin D and the consequent risk of the development of rickets. Although this sequence was very common at the turn of the century, especially in inner urban northern areas, it now occurs in Britain in only a few subgroups of the population—high risk being associated with (a) a vegan diet; (b) a diet high in phytate (a chemical which combines with calcium in the gut preventing its absorption); (c) a pigmented skin. Thus Rastafarians [positive for (a) and (c)] and children of Indo-Pakistani origin [(b) and (c)] are at very high risk and warrant screening for this deficiency and dietary supplementation.

Pollution

In the decades prior to the 1956 Clean Air Act when smog (a combination of fog and air polluted by smoke) was so common in the major cities, there was a strong correlation between air pollution and lower respiratory illness. Indeed the first British national cohort study of children born in 1946 showed that children born in areas of high atmospheric pollution were more liable to lower respiratory infections: the higher the pollution level, the more often and the more severe the infection. The association was found for both upper and lower social classes (Golding 1986). Interestingly there was no such association for upper respiratory infections.

More recent studies have examined associations of particular components of air pollution. There is some evidence, for example, that high levels of ozone are associated with airway resistance (asthmatic-like symptoms) in schoolchildren, high sulphur dioxide levels with increased prevalence of coughing in children and high levels of the oxides of nitrogen with acute respiratory illness.

There are more consistent data, however, to support the contention that indoor air pollution is currently far more important than external pollution. The major sources are smoking adults, gas cookers, and inadequately ventilated heating systems. There is now consistent evidence for a small association between gas cooking and both lower respiratory infection and reduced lung function, thought to be related to the ambient level of nitrogen dioxide. There is stronger evidence of an association between passive smoking (inhalation of tobacco smoke originating from someone else) and childhood respiratory problems, whether measured in terms of pneumonia, bronchitis, pulmonary function, or habitual mouth breathing. Exposure to parental smoking is associated with a deficit over time in the growth of forced vital capacity (a measure of lung function based on the amount of air which can be expelled after a deep breath). That these effects have implications for the future adult is equally demonstrable. A history of lower respiratory illness in early childhood increases the risk of adult chronic respiratory problems (Douglas and Waller 1966).

Whilst such effects should not be ignored, their impact does not compare with other psychological knock-on effects of parental smoking, namely the likelihood that children of smokers will themselves tend to become smokers, the adverse effect of maternal smoking on the fetus, and the psychosocial consequences of parental smoking.

Cigarette smoke contains tar and nicotine but it is not so widely known that it also contains a form of cyanide, the chronic poison carbon monoxide, a radioactive isotope of polonium, and traces of insecticides such as DDT. These are all able to cross the placenta and may affect the fetus. Although observational epidemiological studies are, by their nature, unable to prove causation they suggest that mothers who smoke are more likely to have a perinatal death, a sudden infant death, a growth-retarded infant, or a pre-term delivery and that these associations are not wholly explained by social conditions.

Radiation

Abdominal X-rays in pregnancy may increase the risk that the child will subsequently develop leukaemia but any risk that exists is very small. Whether there is a similar small risk inherent in living near a nuclear power station is still being debated. There are certainly a few small areas near power stations where there are more cases of childhood leukaemia than expected. The suggestion has been made that the risk amounts to one extra case of childhood leukaemia per 60 000 children per year over and above the expected number of two cases per 60 000 children per year (Roman, Beral, Carpenter, Watson, Barton, Ryder, and Aston 1987). Similar clustering has been described however, in many areas that are nowhere near nuclear power stations.

Natural radiation levels are usually higher than those produced by man-made hazards, especially in parts of west Cornwall. The major natural radiation occurs as radon and its so-called daughters which are found in soils and building materials. The walls of a house may emanate these daughter products and the radiation levels may increase substantially when doors and windows are closed. If attached to particles they can be breathed in and absorbed by the body. This is especially likely to happen if there is a smoker in the household, since smoke particles are ideal vehicles. How many cases of childhood cancer may be attributed to such an association is unknown. There has been no research to assess the relationship with passive smoking, although there is some evidence linking childhood cancer with maternal smoking during pregnancy.

Trace metals

Lead has long been known as a poison but debate surrounds the question of the relative toxicity of low levels of lead. In Britain the highest levels of lead are found in soft-water areas, especially when the plumbing is of lead and the family habitually drink the first draw of water. There are also contributions from food and from the exhaust fumes of motor vehicles. The small child is especially prone to ingesting dirt and dust or peeling paint, all of which may contain high lead levels. Controversy has raged over whether relatively high ingestion of lead is causally associated with low intelligence or behaviour problems. The balance of evidence currently favours an association between lead and IQ such that the higher the blood lead level the lower the child's IQ. A partial solution is possible. The blood lead levels in children who wash their hands before eating are, on average, considerably lower than those of children who do not wash their hands. The major thrust in prevention, however, must be to reduce the overall amount of lead in the environment.

Other trace elements such as mercury and cadmium may also be associated with reduced IQ, but information on this is scarce.

Deficiencies of essential trace elements are potentially of greater import. Selenium deficiency in parts of China is known to be responsible for childhood deaths due to a fatal heart condition (Keshan disease). There have been a number of unavailing attempts to identify a link between selenium deficiency and sudden infant death.

Mild zinc deficiency and iron-deficiency anaemia are probably more relevant to contemporary British children. The extreme form of zinc deficiency with dwarfism and hypogonadism (under-developed sex organs) found in the Middle East is not seen here but mild zinc deficiency is probably common and is reportedly associated with childhood diarrhoea, anorexia (loss of appetite), jitteriness, eczematous dermatitis, and depression. Since measurements of zinc status are very difficult, proof of such statements must await prophylactic intervention studies (studies which provide evidence based on administering a substance to a group to see if it will prevent an outcome suspected to be due to deficiency of the substance).

Fluoride

It was suggested as long ago as 1892 that a reason for the increasing frequency of dental caries (decay) could be the relative lack of fluoride consumed by the population. Subsequent population epidemiological studies together with intervention results have proved conclusively that a level of one part per million of fluoride results in a lower incidence of dental caries.

There is no evidence that within Britain or North America the fluoridation of the water supply causes any harmful effects. Thus the potential for preventing the discomfort, morbidity, and expense of having a population with carious teeth is clear. The evidence is unequivocal, yet, except in a few areas, fluoridation has not taken place. It is right that medical recommendations should not be blindly obeyed by the general population and perhaps it is wrong to expect a population fully to appreciate scientific arguments. Nevertheless, the evidence is obvious and, if presented in a clear way, should surely result in a swing of public opinion. There is some urgency in conveying the message to the rest of the world. In many Third World countries the rate of dental decay is increasing rapidly and already exceeds that found in many Western countries.

Other pollutants

Man is naturally an experimenter and is forever producing new food stuffs, new food additives (to preserve food and to make it more attractive), and other chemicals which, while not ostensibly part of the food, are ingested. Such research as has been carried out into the effects of these substances on the child is constantly being superceded by the advent of new substances. What effects there might be on the fetus *in utero* are unknown, but information on the breast-fed infant can be revealing.

It has been shown that an enormous number of substances are excreted in the breast milk, including nicotine, metabolites (break-down products) of drugs the mother may have taken, as well as the chemicals from the foodstuffs themselves. Anecdotes of mothers whose screaming breast-fed babies became placid only after the mother stopped ingesting citrus fruits, Guinness, eggs, coffee, etc. are legion. More scientifically, an interesting study from New Zealand showed that the more varied the maternal diet the more likely the baby was to have 'colic'.

More threatening, however, is the story of the polychlorinated and polybrominated biphenyls (PCB and PBB). These chemicals are used in various industrial processes and are pollutants that can contaminate the soil, vegetation, and water supply. They are not biodegradable (do not break down naturally) but can enter the food chain when consumed (e.g. by a cow eating the vegetation or a fish swallowing water). There are mechanisms for storing these substances within the body but none for excreting them in either man or mammal, other than through breast milk. Isolated incidents involving infants which have resulted in excessive intake have resulted in severe neurological abnormalities. There is now some evidence, however, that milder doses may also have adverse effects on IQ and child development especially when inadvertent ingestion has occurred in pregnancy (Golding 1986).

Housing

There is little consistant evidence that good housing contributes to health. Areas with poor housing will lack amenities such as running hot water or baths. Areas with overcrowded households tend to have higher mortality rates for children under five years of age, but not for older children. If one considers the actual house in which a child lives, however, evidence for a detrimental effect is confusing. For children born in 1946 an association was found between overcrowding and early bronchitis or pneumonia, but for those born in 1958 no such adverse health effect of overcrowding could be found (Golding, 1986).

Heating is an obvious component of housing and it might be thought that new centrally heated homes would have an obvious advantage, especially in terms of respiratory problems. In South Wales, a population study of respiratory illness was undertaken among children from three areas with different types of housing (a) new centrally heated council houses; (b) council houses with open coal fires; (c) traditional older houses with open fires. Compared with the rest of the sample, children living in the new centrally heated houses had a higher incidence of colds and reduced lung function. The children least at risk were those living in the traditional older houses. They had fewer sore throats and colds, and generally better lung function.

Water supply

In the 1960s it was first shown that within England and Wales adult mortality rates were higher in soft-water areas than in hard-water areas (Gardner, Crawford, and Morris 1969). Subsequent studies have shown that this was also true of infant mortality in Britain (Crawford, Gardner, and Sedgwick 1972) but not in the USA (Spiers, Wright, and Siegel 1974).

Residents of soft-water areas have been shown to excrete higher levels of sodium (largely due to the fact that they seem to put more salt on their food) and to have elevated lead levels in both blood and bone.

An inadvertant experiment concerning the importance of softness of the water in determining the blood lead level occurred in Glasgow when the water was artificially hardened. Mothers in the maternity hospital were subsequently found to have substantially lower blood lead levels (Moore, Goldberg, Morton Fyfe, and Richards 1981).

Should it be recommended that all soft-water supplies be hardened at source? Where there are lead pipes or storage tanks this seems sensible since soft acid water will dissolve some of the lead; it cannot be deduced, however, that such a procedure would necessarily reduce the infant mortality rate. In hard-water areas, many homes and hospitals use artificial softeners. Although this might make washing easier, there is some evidence that it may be harmful to health. Water softening increases the concentration of sodium ions in the water with an increased risk of hypernatraemia (excessive sodium in the blood) in the young infant and possibly hypertension (increased blood pressure) in childhood.

Nutrition

The yearly reports '*The state of the world's children*' published by the World Health Organization and the United Nations International Children's Emergency Fund highlight the continuing problems of undernutrition and infection which so erode the health of many of the children in the world. British paediatricians have a tradition of involvement with these problems overseas, both in practice and in research. For many children in the developing world where food means survival the nutritional concerns and controversies of the UK seem sadly irrelevant. Recent surveys suggest that most children in the UK today are well fed. Nevertheless, there is good reason to think that simpler and more judicious eating would improve their health.

Milk

The first recommendation of the Department of Health and Social Security Report '*Present Day Practice in Infant Feeding*' (DHSS 1974) was that breast-feeding should be encouraged. Very few would doubt that for all but a small minority of infants human milk is the best and that we should do all we can to encourage and support mothers who wish to breast-feed.

Human milk is a complete nutrient for most human infants; breast-feeding also has psychological merits beyond the value of the food, yet many parents still elect to bottle-feed their infants with an artificial feed. It is some encouragement, however, that at a time when the percentage of working mothers and single parent families is on the increase, the percentage of mothers breast-feeding is not falling (Martin and Monk 1982).

In the absence of any objective evidence, DHSS (1981) recommends that infant artificial feeds should resemble 'average' human milk in as far as that is technically possible. At present that means that the energy content and the amounts of protein, carbohydrate, fat, minerals and vitamins are of the same order. But there are still differences in the nature of the carbohydrate, fat, and especially protein. Differences in carbohydrate (lactose or glucose syrup) or fat (low or moderate proportions of unsaturated fatty acids) may well be of little moment. The differences in proteins are considerable and may be important. Both the curds and whey protein of cow's milk are very different from the curds and whey in human milk. The whey fraction in human milk contains IgA, lactoferrin, and isoenzymes which together may well be the components which provide the infant bowel with some protection against infection: they hardly figure in the whey protein of cow's milk. It is the cow's milk whey fraction B lactoalbumin, however, which may be the most allergenic constituent. This is only found in human milk in trace amounts at the most if the mother eats milk products.

The manufacturing companies will no doubt continue to use new technical developments to improve artificial feeds to the benefit of infants. Each 'advance' presents nutritional experts, paediatricians and regulatory bodies with difficult decisions. Current issues include the need or desirability of adding substances found in human milk such as carnitine, nucleotides, or lactoferrin, or others, to the feed.

The nutritional advantages of human milk have been well rehearsed in the last few years, and there is a risk in overstating the benefits, but by the same token there is also a risk in underestimating the persuasive power of the promotion of artificial feeds.

After milk

The second recommendation of the report, Infant Feeding 1980 (Martin and Monk 1982) was that the introduction of solid foods should be delayed until four to six months. Although there has been some improvement, 80 per cent of British infants in 1980 were being offered solid food by four months of age. The initial solid feeds are now mainly based on maize and rice, all gluten free (a type of protein which in a few infants causes coeliac disease), which, with the increasing incidence of breast-feeding, may be responsible for the apparent decline in the numbers of British children suffering from coeliac disease.

As the array of liquid milk products—half-skimmed, skimmed, fortified, etc.—increases, so each age group will be presented with a selection of tins and bottles specially designed with their nutritional requirements in mind. Will the choice be an improvement?

What is good for the majority of weaning infants will not be appropriate for some. Problems will continue to arise amongst those who differ by virtue of wealth (or lack of it), capability, geography, culture, as well as individual idiosyncracy. Vigilance is required, particularly over the weaning periods for those who are missing out. Seeking out infants with nutritional deficiencies resulting in failure to thrive, iron deficiency anaemia, or rickets is the task of the community paediatric team.

Are all British children getting enough to eat?

Even in a country where food is plentiful it is still important to ask the question, 'Are *all* the children getting enough to eat?' Oppe (1980) has said that the desired goal of a national nutritional strategy is that every child is offered a diet that is conducive to normal health, growth, and development and which will best enable him or her to avoid nutritionally related disease in adult life. That is quite a tall order. National policies can only be based on appropriate information; what might that be in the context of the defined objective?

In this country now, undernutrition is unlikely to have a detectable impact on mortality rates, but might it affect growth? Over the last century children have been growing faster, maturing earlier, and reaching an increased adult height (DHSS 1978). No doubt this is due to many factors including better nutrition. The trend seems to be slowing down suggesting that the better conditions have now had their maximal impact. It cannot be assumed, however, that growing faster, maturing earlier, and being taller are necessarily associated with a long and happy life. They came at a time of affluence, and they may be associated with the diseases of affluence: obesity, heart attacks late-onset diabetes, etc.

There still is, and always has been, a difference in the mean adult height in different social classes. In surveys conducted in the 1930s it was found that children aged 10 to 16 years in fee-paying schools were on average taller than those at grammar schools who were in turn taller than those in council schools or those who were working and had left school at 14 years of age (DHSS 1978). In the Newcastle study (1947–1962) these differences were present at four years of age and increased as the child grew older (Miller, Court, Knox, and Brandon 1974). Whilst accepting that adult height is determined in part by genetic make-up and in part by many environmental influences, it still seems reasonable to work on the assumption that if all children were to enjoy the best possible diet the variation in average height and weight between different socio-economic groups in Britain would be less marked.

In the 1920s Dr Corry Mann showed that orphan boys who drank a pint of milk a day became lively and grew faster. In 1940 when food was short in the Second World War, all schoolchildren were offered one-third of a pint of milk daily, a practice which was continued until 1968. It was difficult at the time to think it did anything but good and it is difficult now to find any evidence that it did any harm. After it was withdrawn from secondary schools in 1968 it was found that those children on a marginal diet in South Wales did grow taller if given a milk supplement (Baker, Elwood, Hughes, Jones, Moore, and Sweetman 1980). The 1980 Education Act permitted, but did not require, local authorities to provide free school milk for children in nursery and primary education and special schools.

In 1982 an EEC scheme was introduced so that local authorities could claim substantial subsidies on milk and milk products used in schools, including flavoured semi-skimmed milks and yoghurts. Hopefully a morning snack nutrient-rich in protein, calcium, and riboflavin will be on offer for all schoolchildren. This may be particularly important for those who miss their breakfast (5–10 years, 8 per cent; 10–14 years, 13 per cent; 14–18 years, 20 per cent), although there is no evidence that going to school on an empty stomach affects performance (Dickie and Bender 1982).

Prior to 1980, local authorities were obliged to provide school meals for all schoolchildren with the intention that these meals should provide 33 per cent of the energy and 42 per cent of the protein of the recommended daily amount. In practice they often fell short. School meals make an important contribution to the nutrient intake of some schoolchildren, and yet under the 1980 Education Act local authorities are only *required* to provide school meals for the children of parents on supplementary benefit. School meals are appreciated by a majority of children; they have social and educational value and can be made attractive with cash cafeteria systems so that the recommended amounts are achieved.

If there is any truth in the assertion that weight is an index of short-term and height of long-term food intake, then perhaps that information should be collected in a precise and informed manner by the community paediatric service to identify those children who might be thin or stunted through lack of sufficient food. To guide national policy on food supplements, there is a need not only for ongoing studies like the National Food Family Expenditure Survey, but also to establish a national programme for the regular and routine collection of anthropometric (measurement of body size and proportions) data from large representative samples of British children (Oppe 1980).

Are British children eating the right foods?
When food is plentiful, it is the choice which creates difficulties and excesses become a problem. The choice is becoming more bewildering now that food manufacturing technology is such that 'novel' vegetable protein can be made to resemble meat, milk shakes can taste of many fruits, potato crisps of many savouries, and most foods can be stored, preserved, and coloured so that they are available and appear fresh throughout the year. Sales promotion has ensured that a brown, sweet, fizzy drink is thought desirable by many children in the world. So, we must be on our guard. Appealing fast foods may do harm, they may even do good, but it seems unlikely that they will make no difference. Perhaps their impact will be more on the social activity of eating together, in families and in groups, than on our children's nutritional status. Nevertheless, pesticides and chemicals on the farm and colouring

and preservatives in food manufacture can harm vulnerable children. Protecting children from inappropriate foods is a responsibility shared by parents and the government bodies which can exert control on industry. Guiding children to establish sensible eating habits is a responsibility parents share with the Health Educational Council, the British Nutrition Foundation, and those who determine the school curriculum, amongst others.

It falls to the doctor, often the paediatrician, to decide whether one or other food is detrimental to the health of the individual child. In the past the nutritional expertise of paediatricians has been largely confined to feeding problems in infancy like vomiting and regurgitation, failure to thrive, post-gastro-enteritis intolerances, coeliac disease, and the dietary management of cystic fibrosis, phenylketonuria (see p. 266), and other metabolic disorders. However, now that it is alleged that there is a nutritional component in many of the common childhood disorders, like asthma, eczema, recurrent headaches, and hyperactivity, and that many of the common adult diseases, like obesity, late-onset diabetes, hypertension, heart attacks, schizophrenia, and some cancers, have their origin, in part, in early eating patterns, paediatricians are being asked to resolve more difficult problems, and for the forseeable future these problems are unlikely to become easier.

Two complex issues, the development of obesity and the effect of additives on behaviour, have been the subject of many studies over the last decade. It appears that early over-feeding does not have the permanent impact on adult shape that was originally suggested, that fat children do not necessarily become fat adults (Braddon, Rodgers, Wadsworth, and Davies 1986), and that sensible eating will help some children to avoid becoming overweight—but the real pathogenesis of obesity remains an enigma. By contrast certain chemicals in minute amounts do seem to be specific poisons to individual children, and to disturb their behaviour; however, the degree and extent of such effects has yet to be defined. But all children are not the same; some will be more at risk than others and it is the identification and counselling of those families at risk which will increasingly fall to paediatricians. Do paediatricians know enough about nutrition to be able to do this? This is but one reason why the recommendations of the British Nutrition Foundation on improving the nutrition education content of the medical syllabus should be supported.

Infection

A century ago, less than 60 per cent of children survived to five years of age, now over 98 per cent do so. The difference is largely due to the control of infections. By the 1940s, before antibiotics and vaccines were widely used, the mortality rate had already fallen due to better nutrition and a cleaner environment. Nevertheless, infection was still a major hazard, children's hospitals were designed with small separated ward areas and plenty of isolation cubicles, and visiting was not encouraged because of the risk of cross-infection. A houseman on paediatric wards in the 1950s would see many children with chronic sepsis, mastoiditis (infection of the mastoid bone associated with an infected ear), bronchiectasis (lungs damaged by infection), osteomyelitis (infection of bone), and prolonged illness due to rheumatic fever and acute nephritis. Tuberculosis was common and it was routine to perform a tuberculin test on every child admitted; special ward areas were designated for gastro-enteritis which was frequently fatal; and the children with obvious 'infectious diseases' like poliomyelitis, diphtheria, and whooping cough were immediately transferred to infectious disease hospitals. Over the 1940s and 1950s, effective antibiotics became widely available and national vaccination programmes were introduced. Now most of the diseases listed above are rare, children with infections are nursed in general paediatric wards, and epidemics are not feared in the way they were. We run the risk of forgetting, however, that although mortality from certain childhood infections has fallen, infections are *still* a major health problem and are likely to remain so.

Babies are born sterile into a world containing many micro-organisms which can invade and infect the body and, if they are not overcome, cause permanent damage or death. The factors controlling the numbers, nature, and infectivity of these organisms are ill understood. Many infections are being reported less, like tuberculosis, but others are increasing like those due to campylobacteria, chlamydia, and cryptococci. Even more disturbing are the appearances of apparently new infections like Legionnaires' disease and AIDS. Fortunately, the numbers at present are few but are unlikely to remain that way.

Vaccination

Paediatricians have the dual responsibility of being aware of the changing 'micro-organism' environment and taking whatever steps are necessary to protect children when they experience infections. Universal good health, reduced exposure by virtue of environmental improvements, and early treatment with effective antibacterial and antiviral agents should reduce the risks of infection further, but it is unrealistic to expect a world free of pathogens. The alternative strategy of controlled exposure to vaccines, so that children build up resistance to the pathogens they are likely to meet, currently offers the most sure way of protecting them through childhood.

At present infants experience many infections as a matter of chance. The development of more and more vaccines brings with it the opportunity of the controlled development of the body's defences.

Vaccination programmes are designed not only to benefit individuals but to develop community immunity as well. The world strategy for smallpox vaccination appears to have eradicated the organism as a pathogen in man. Whooping cough infection is said to be virtually eradicated in Hungary and measles in the USA. In Britain the incidence of whooping cough continued to fall with the introduction of the national vaccination programme in 1957 but subsequently increased when the vaccination uptake rate fell to below 50 per cent. The fall in uptake arose from concern, probably misplaced, that the vaccine itself might cause brain damage or death and resulted in a considerable proportion of older children being unprotected. It is young infants, however, who are most vulnerable to whooping cough and they are now more at risk because their older unimmunized brothers and sisters may bring whooping cough home. A protected family protects the baby.

There is a strong argument for an agreed approach to vaccination within a population, but this raises many difficult issues. There can be no common template in that there are differences in the epidemiology of each disease within populations; causative organisms differ in behaviour potency; vaccines have different modes of action. Each infection has to be considered separately. Furthermore the epidemiology and the actual and perceived need of the vaccine are continually changing.

Every vaccine that is pronounced efficacious and safe on the recommendation of the Committee on Safety of Medicines will still have a risk as well as a benefit. An informed decision can only be made after an analysis of all the benefits and risks and a recognition of who gets the benefit and who takes the risk. For individuals, age groups, and selected populations, the balance of benefit and risk is still not known. For example, should infants with residual neurological problems following a birth event be vaccinated against pertussis (whooping cough). In France, the experts say yes, whilst in Britain the expert view is cautious. There is currently little evidence to support either view. In the 1950s many children died of diphtheria; yet an effective and safe vaccine was available. Many are dying of measles now; yet there are effective vaccines offered and available free. It is the role of paediatricians to explain the potential benefits and the balance of benefit and risk. The British Paediatric Association Immunization and Vaccine Advisory Committee supports the early introduction of the combined measles, mumps, rubella vaccine (MMR).

New vaccines   The most successful vaccines have been those concerned with epidemic infections which often cause death or severe damage, like diptheria and polio. Measles and pertussis are highly infectious and may be dangerous, so nearly everyone receiving the injection can expect to benefit. The same would be true for vaccines against rotavirus (which is one cause of gastro-enteritis) or respiratory syncytial virus (which causes chest infection particularly in babies). Paediatricians would be concerned to achieve good post-market surveillance should such vaccines become available. It is in the area of rare disorders that the issues become more complex. Rubella (German measles) vaccine was introduced to avoid a rare but severe embryopathy (damage to the embryo *in utero*). Vaccines against pneumococcal and haemophilus influenzae infections are available but little used. Meningitis from these organisms still occurs and is lethal in a few (approximately 5 per cent) and causes permanent brain damage in some (approximately 10 per cent). Earlier diagnosis and treatment may improve the figures. These are clinical matters on which paediatricians are required to make judgements.

Continuing problems
Respiratory illnesses are still the commonest affliction of children, causing them to miss school, attend doctors, receive antibiotics, analgesics, and antipyretics, become deaf, and undergo operations such as tonsillectomy, adenoidectomy, or myringotomy (incision of the ear-drum when the middle ear is infected). There is substantial

evidence that childhood respiratory infections predispose to chronic airways disease in adults. Even if an effective vaccine or antiviral agent becomes available against the main epidemic respiratory disease, bronchiolitis (affecting infants particularly), many problems will remain.

Social environment

Social class

It is generally assumed that a social class variation in morbidity implies an association with physical or social deprivation. The social class definitions used in this country take no account of deprivation at all—and are based on a classification of the occupation of the head of the household (usually the father of the child). Substantial jusification for this is found in the perinatal (stillbirths plus first-week death) and infant mortality (deaths in the first year of life) statistics where there is always a dramatic trend over the six categories (I, II, III non-manual, III manual, IV, and V) with lowest mortality in social class I (the higher professionals—doctors, ministers of religion, solicitors, etc.) and highest mortality in social class V (cleaners, labourers). That the classification is not synonymous with income is obvious (social class II includes teachers and nurses who are relatively poorly paid compared with III manual, the craftsmen and other skilled manual workers), yet the trend in mortality persists.

One of the challenges of epidemiology is to tease out the component parts of a social class trend. Factors that have been shown to vary with social class include the education of the parents, their smoking habits, their use of health-care services (such as contraception, immunization, antenatal care), diet, breast-feeding, the number of children in the household, type of housing, and so on.

Such studies that have successfully attempted to ascertain the variables responsible for social class trends have shown, for example, that the overall trend in mean birth-weight is 'explained' by the fact that mothers in the 'lower' social classes are physically shorter and more likely to smoke. An association with wheezing attacks can be shown to be due to greater prevalence of maternal smoking; repeated childhood accidents are secondary to the type of area in which a family lives. Other trends in social class that have yet to be totally explained in terms of component parts include associations with bed-wetting, temper tantrums, headaches and bronchitis. Some or all of these conditions may well be related to family discord, disruption, and stress.

Persisting adversities

There is a general assumption that children must be affected by their upbringing and that 'bad' experiences in early life inevitably damage a child's psychological development. Yet it is clear that the link between adverse experiences and emotional or behavioural problems is far from straightforward. In the first instance, some of the associations are mediated genetically rather than environmentally. Children and their parents share genes, and in some cases effects that appear environmental are partly hereditary. For example, intelligent parents tend to have more intelligent children, a link that is a consequence of both biological inheritance and experience in growing up. A second consideration is that children are not passive recipients of environmental input. They engage with their environment in an active fashion, *eliciting* behaviour from others and shaping their experiences both by their influences on interpersonal interactions and by their *choice* of situations. The constitutionally outgoing child is likely to choose to engage in more social encounters but, by so doing, will be exposed to more social experiences that will in turn serve to shape his development. A third point is that people vary greatly in their response to bad experiences. Some succumb with serious psychiatric problems, some have only minor temporary difficulties in adjustment, others escape relatively unscathed, and a few may actually be strengthened by having coped successfully with hazards and difficulties. The last is not as surprising as it seems at first sight. After all, immunization provides protection by exposure to the germs and not by their avoidance or by the promotion of positive physical health. The exposure is protective because the infectious agent has been modified so that the 'mini-infection' is well within the body's scope to deal with successfully. Probably the same applies to psychosocial stresses.

Risks and resiliences

A further consideration is that children go on developing. Adverse experiences do not permanently damage personalities. Of course, like physical injuries, they leave scars and vulnerabilities but most of the long-term effects are indirect, rather than direct. That is, there are chain reactions in which the immediate impact of adversities leads to behaviour that makes more bad experiences likely or which causes children to react in ways that are maladaptive and damaging. But the chains can be broken if later experiences are sufficiently beneficial.

In recent years attention has come to be focused on turning points in people's lives when good experiences can alter a risk trajectory on to a more adaptive path. Good relationships and the experience of some form of success are both important in this connection, probably because they serve to change the ways in which people think about themselves and their environment. Good functioning is aided by high self-esteem (the feeling that you are a worthy person) and self-efficacy (the confidence that you can cope with challenges). It is interesting and important that these potential turning points can arise quite late in the development process. For example, a successful, harmonious marriage can do much to counter the ill effects of an unhappy upbringing.

At one time childhood adversities tended to be grouped together under the general heading of 'maternal deprivation'. It is now appreciated that this was rather misleading because the experiences are heterogeneous, with different forms of adversity having different effects. Thus the mother is not the only person of importance to children (Rutter 1981). Damage can often come either from the harmful happenings to which children are exposed or from deprivation of the good experiences which other children experience. Nevertheless, the original concept has proved correct in its emphasis on the important role of children's early relationships within the family (Bowlby 1969). Ordinarily, children develop close selective attachments which serve to provide love and security and which go on to help form the basis of other relationships, both friendships and love relationships. Human beings are social animals and right throughout life intimate relationships provide protection; their loss (through bereavement, divorce, or rebuff) creates a serious stress.

In the study of environmental risks, it is always necessary to proceed from risk *indicators* to risk *mechanisms*. In other words one usually starts from an observation that an association with some broad variable (such as poor living conditions) is accompanied by an increased risk of some disease or disorder. It is then necessary to go on to determine just *which* aspect of that variable is responsible for the process that leads to the undesirable outcome. Sometimes animal experiments help. For example, these have been important in showing that the separation of an infant from parents tends to be damaging because it leads to harmful patterns of parent-infant interactions following reunion. More often, however, it is necessary to search for 'natural' experiments that provide the appropriate contrasts to test different causal hypotheses. Thus the comparison of unhappy separations (as with family break-up) and happy ones (as with holidays or staying with friends or relatives) shows that the fact of children being apart from their families tends to be less important than the circumstances that follow, precede, and occur during the separation. Stressful separations, however (as with parental divorce), may add to children's difficulties.

Fostering, adoption, and institutional rearing

These issues are very pertinent in the consideration of atypical patterns of rearing. Society often has to face the issue that children may have to be compulsorily removed from their parents because of neglect or maltreatment. The dangers from physical child abuse are plain to see but the risks associated with emotional neglect or psychological abuse may be just as great. The decision on when to intervene has to be influenced not only by the risks to the child from remaining in the home but also from the quality of the alternatives that are available. Residential nurseries and children's homes are not very satisfactory places in which to grow up. In them, although it is often possible to ensure that children have a wide and interesting range of experiences, that there is plenty of talk and play, that relationships with staff are good, and that the physical environment is of a good quality, it is much more difficult is to provide continuity in care-giving. Children in institutions may have as many as 50 people looking after them over the course of a few years. Follow-up studies to adult life of young people who have been brought up in children's homes have shown that many suffer, although some do well. The marked discontinuity in relationships may be the damaging factor (Rutter 1987*a*).

Foster families have been seen as a better alternative and indeed the limited available evidence suggests that they are. Nevertheless, again it has proved difficult to provide adequate security of relationships. All too often, strains in the foster family, or practical difficulties, lead to children having to change families. A pillar-to-post upbringing is not helpful. Adoption provides a solution for some. For children from seriously disturbed backgrounds this can reduce the psychological risks, even when adoption does not take place until quite late. Adopted children reared in advantaged homes develop well on the whole, with intellectual qualities that are at least average (Rutter 1981). For the most part, they also have a good outcome in terms of their socio-emotional development. Nevertheless, the risks of problems are greater than normal, perhaps especially in adolescence. These may stem from uncertainties about being 'different'. When properly handled, such uncertainties are easily managed but when not well dealt with, or when children are constitutionally more vulnerable, problems may arise. Psychological manipulations may well bring benefits but, just as with powerful medications, the benefits tend to be accompanied by the risk of undesirable side-effects. It is important to get the balance right.

Parental mental disorders

It has long been known that parental mental disorder increases the risk that the children will suffer psychiatric problems but it has been less clear which factors were mainly responsible for the risk. Several different mechanisms are important (Rutter 1987*b*). The main hazards do not derive from the manifestations of the mental disorder as such, although these may be important if they directly impinge on the children in some way. Rather the family discord often associated with psychiatric disorder in parents constitutes the commonest risk feature, with the risks greatest when parental irritability or hostility focuses on one scapegoat child. In addition, however, it is apparent that severe mental disorders may distort parenting in ways that interfere with secure parent–child relationships. Family break-up may bring further stresses.

The risks associated with parental mental disorder do not derive only from psychological disturbances in the family; there are also physical and developmental risks. For example, alcohol ingestion by the mother may damage her child's brain because alcohol in the mother's blood passes to the embryo and causes interference with the developmental process. It is not known what amount of alcohol consumption is safe in pregnancy but it is evident that the risks are present at drinking levels well below drunkenness. It is important to inform people of the damage to the baby that may stem from alcohol, drugs, and smoking in pregnancy. Equally, children may be harmed by the disruptions and distortions in child-rearing associated with parental alcoholism.

With some serious mental disorders such as schizophrenia there are also genetic risks (we know that this is so because there is an increased risk of schizophrenia in children born to schizophrenic mothers but adopted by healthy parents). The disorders in the children are not inherited directly but there is a substantially increased vulnerability to the particular abnormalities associated with schizophrenia.

Family discord and disruption

Serious discord and quarrelling in families predispose children to emotional and behavioural problems. This is so for children of all ages although the particular ways in which young people react varies with their phase of development. On the whole, boys seem to suffer more than girls, although both sexes are at risk. The risks seem greatest when children are brought into parental quarrels and when children get picked on systematically. Vicious circles of interaction readily develop in which the children respond to the discord by becoming difficult themselves, which further serves to irritate the parents who then react in ways that prolong the tension and hostility.

Persistent family conflict is seriously unsettling to children and it is important to appreciate the extent to which even very young children are affected. A restoration of family harmony makes it more likely that children will develop normally but, if discord is prolonged, children's problems may become so established that to some extent they are self-perpetuating unless active steps are taken to help them. While parental divorces may be the best available solution when parents cannot maintain a reasonable degree of family cohesion in spite of strenuous efforts to do so, the break-up of the family presents new stresses for the child and all too often parental disputes (over finances, access, and the like) continue long after the divorce. It seems that, on average, it takes most people some two years to get back on an even keel following divorce, but it can take much longer. Parental remarriage, if the marriage is a happy one, usually improves the situation (both emotional and financial) for the adults involved. However, things are more complicated for the children, with problems especially common between stepfathers and daughters. Boys, on the other hand, can benefit from the presence of a responsive parent of the same sex who can provide authoritative support for both the mother and son.

Acute psychosocial stresses

During recent years increasing attention has come to be paid to the role of acutely stressful life events as precipitants of physical and psychiatric disorder, especially depression, in adults. Ill-effects seem most likely when the acute events either bring about long-term changes in patterns of life (as occurs with bereavement, divorce, or loss of a job) or carry long-term threats to people's views of themselves (as with a humiliating rebuff or public failure). There is more limited evidence on effects on childhood but much the same seems to occur. However, there are some important differences. It is clear that the impact of unpleasant experiences is mediated in large part by what people *think* about what has happened to them. Children's powers of conceptualization are more limited than those of adults and this limitation may either protect them or put them more at risk. For example, young babies are less distressed than toddlers by admission to hospital because they have yet to develop strong attachments that could be disrupted by admission and because they do not possess the ability to experience *anticipatory* fear. On the other hand, toddlers are more often adversely affected than school-age children because older children have a capacity lacked by pre-schoolers to maintain relationships during a period of absence and to understand what events such as hospital admission are all about.

A second difference from adults, at least in emphasis, is the importance for children of the effects of events on their patterns of interaction with other people. A birth of a younger brother or sister constitutes a very common 'normal' life stress because the older child has to cope with a rival for the parents' affection and attention. Jealousy between siblings can be surprisingly long-lasting and in some instances may form the core of an emotional disorder. There are immense variations between children in how far this is a problem. Much of a variation is explicable in terms of the effects on patterns of family interaction. Difficulties are more likely when the arrival of the new baby results in a marked diminution in the amount of parental time spent with the first-born; when parents become more demanding of the older child; and when parents respond negatively to the first-born's jealousy of the baby and to his confrontational demands that attention be paid to him. With all age groups long-term sequelae tend to be influenced by interaction and chain effects of various kinds. For example, a single hospital admission rarely leads to a persisting emotional disorder but multiple admissions are more likely to do so, especially if they are accompanied by chronic family adversities. Similarly, parental loss is most likely to create a persistent vulnerability if it is followed by a loss of affectionate parental care, because the remaining parent reacts badly to the loss, or because family resources are inadequate (Brown, Harris, and Bifulco 1986; Rutter 1987*a*).

The different ways in which the ill-effects of acute stresses may be ameliorated are well illustrated by the findings on hospital admission. The first approach is through steps to alter the stress itself. One of the stressful aspects of admission for young children is the separation from the family. Facilities to allow one parent to stay overnight with the child have made an important difference in that connection, as has unrestricted visiting. Boredom and confinement to bed provide a different kind of stress, one that has been reduced by play and educational provision in hospitals. Steps to reduce the unpleasantness of medical and surgical procedure have also been of benefit. The second approach is to alter children's attitudes to hospital so that they are better able to cope with the experience. The prior experience of separations in happy circumstances (as through familiar baby-sitters and staying overnight with friends and relatives) helps, as do programmes to prepare children for hospital (just before they are due to go in for a planned admission). Although not adequately tested, it is likely that a third approach, namely altering the consequencies of the experience, may also be of benefit. At least in part, longer term sequelae are a function of maladaptive patterns of family interaction that may be set up. It is normal for young children to be either rather clinging or rebuffing of parents on return home and some become more babyish. It may be helpful for parents to appreciate that this is an expected transient response that needs reassurance rather than discipline.

Day care and schooling
During recent years, in many industrialised nations there has been an increase in the proportion of mothers of young children who

have taken jobs outside the home. This has been accompanied by an increase in the number of families who have sought day care of one kind or another for their children. It is a mistake to assume that this is a really new phenomenon as parents all over the world have always made extensive use of non-parental care-givers—as emphasised by the title of Werner's (1983) book on the topic: *Kith, Kin and Hired Hands*. What is new is a widespread concern about whether non-familial day care is good or bad for young children. The findings show that the matter is not a clear-cut cause for alarm or satisfaction (Zigler and Gordon 1982). The experience of day care is neither good nor bad in itself; much depends on its quality. Satisfaction is not warranted, because too much day care falls well short of what is required; alarm is not indicated because most of the faults are remediable without too much difficulty if there is a will to do what is needed. Most of the evidence, however, applies to children over the age of two or three years and recent research has raised questions on whether the effects are so generally benign in the first year of life. Clearly, even very young children usually cope satisfactorily but it may be that group care outside the home is more difficult for some infants if such care starts at a time when they are just beginning to form strong attachments to their parents. On the other hand, there is some evidence that, for children with seriously disadvantaged homes, unusually high-quality day care (with a substantial educational component) at a slightly older age may be protective.

Children spend a high proportion of their waking hours at school between the ages of 5 and 16 years. The main goal of schooling is education but inevitably schooling also provides important social experiences, experiences that can have positive or negative effects. Research findings have been consistent in showing that some schools are much more successful than others in making it possible for children to gain high achievements and to function well socially and emotionally. There is no one 'recipe' for success; the schools that do well for their pupils have quite a range of styles. However, what they tend to have in common is a purposive goal-oriented approach that includes an expectation that children will do well, a sensitivity to the individual needs of children, ample encouragement as part of a positive ethos that is not marred by excessive focus on punishment and good opportunities for all pupils to exercise initiative and responsibility. Less attention has been paid to the

members include paediatricians, paediatric surgeons, general practitioners, community physicians, and nurses as well as representatives from many government departments, voluntary organizations, and professional bodies. Its object is to act as a scientific advisory and co-ordinating body. It functions in two main ways: first by producing reports on specific problems that aim to influence policy, and second through selected educational approaches. It does not produce educational material as this is already being done by the Royal Society for the Prevention of Accidents and the Health Educational Authority, both of which are represented on the Trust. It has a resource centre used by students and researchers and it receives a large number of enquiries from individuals and organizations (Jackson and Gaffin 1983).

Discussion

The environment, taken to mean 'the conditions or influences under which any person or thing lives or is developed', is certainly a major factor influencing the well-being of the modern child. Having accepted this fact, the next step is to consider how the environment may be changed in order to improve the health of the nation's children. Politicians may assume that improving the average wage, housing conditions, or hospital facilities may be the prime need, but just as it is necessary to carry out randomized controlled trials to judge the benefits and hazards of a new therapy scientifically, it is important similarly to evaluate social measures. A consideration of the results of observational studies points to some unexpected conclusions.

For example, since the Second World War, the conditions in which children have been brought up have changed dramatically. In 1950, 45 per cent of households with pre-school children had no bath or shower and 50 per cent had no hot running water. By 1975 the comparable figures were 5 per cent and 6.5 per cent, respectively. Over the same period there was a dramatic decrease in the number of households which were technically overcrowded (6 per cent to 1.8 per cent), and the proportion of households in the upper social classes increased (18.7 per cent to 26.5 per cent). The parental educational levels had also increased (3.7 per cent to 17.1 per cent with university degrees) (Osborn, Butler, and Morris 1985). Yet proof that such dramatic social and environmental improvements were associated with overall reductions in ill health is lacking. Although childhood mortality has fallen largely due to a reduction in the major infections, there is evidence that chronic conditions such as asthma and eczema may be increasing along with child abuse and childhood delinquency. Disabilities which have long been considered to be preventable with improvements in obsetetric and neonatal care, such as cerebral palsy, have shown little sign of diminishing.

How then can we suggest ways that the environment be manipulated? It is pertinent to remember that obvious solutions may have surprising hazards. As sanitary conditions improved this century, paralytic poliomyelitis became increasingly more prevalent with the highest incidences in the upper social classes. Apparently the polio virus has always been endemic prior to the twentieth century, with the population gaining immunity from earliest infancy. As hygiene improved the numbers of children and adults who were susceptible to infection increased, especially in the upper social classes.

The modern family is increasingly under stress and, as we have shown, stress may be associated with physical and psychological morbidity. Stress can rarely be removed—indeed some stress is an important component of life—yet the ability to cope with stress can be improved. In the USA a recent randomized controlled trial showed that by increasing the high-risk mother's social support there was a significant reduction in both child abuse and in childhood accidents. This must await confirmation.

Another way in which the child is influenced without our overt awareness concerns peer pressure. This is an immense influence in persuading a child or adolescent to smoke, drink alcohol, try heroin, or experiment with sex.

Children's attitudes may also be largely influenced by the media, especially television. It is notoriously difficult to document such relationships but two recent American studies (Phillips and Carstensen 1986; Gould and Shaffer 1986) provide disturbing reading: there were significant increases in teenage suicide attempts in the days following news stories or films involving suicide. The association was barely perceptible for adults but marked for adolescents.

If our youngsters are so easily swayed towards suicide by occasional television reports, how much more impression on their vulnerable minds do repeated demonstrations of mugging, marital violence, child sexual abuse, or rape have? If as few as 10 per cent of the present generation of children are affected the consequent problems for the next generation of children must be immense. This insidious pollution of the mind may be a far more potent threat to the present and future generations than the currently prominent anxieties over nuclear reactors, food additives, or inner city decay which, although important, directly affect relatively few children. The way ahead is to generate physically and psychologically balanced and healthy parents, and this can only happen through a change in the current trend of attitudes to the nation's children. Collaboration between the medical and teaching professions, psychologists, and social scientists may help solve some, if not all, the current problems, but it is more likely that the present state of affairs will only improve when society as a whole changes some of its attitudes.

References

Baker, I. A., Elwood, P. C., Hughes, J., Jones, M., Moore, F., and Sweetman, P. (1980). A randomised controlled trial of the effect of the provision of free school milk on the growth of children. *Journal of Epidemiology and Community Health* **34**, p. 31.

Bowlby, J. (1969). *Attachment and loss: I. Attachment* Hogarth Press, London.

Braddon, F. M., Rodgers, B., Wadsworth, M. E. J. and Davies, J. M. C. (1986). Onset of obesity in a 36 year birth cohort study. *British Medical Journal* **293**, pp. 299-303.

Brown, G. W., Harris, T. O., and Bifulco, A. (1986). The long term effects of early loss of parent. In *Depression in young people: clinical and developmental perspectives.* (Eds. M. Rutter, C. C. Izard, and P. B. Read), pp. 251-96. Guildford Press, New York.

Butler, N. R. and Golding, J. (1986), *From birth to five: a study of the health and behaviour of a national cohort.* Pergamon Press, Oxford.

Crawford, M. D., Gardner, M. J., and Sedgwick, P. A. (1972). Infant mortality and hardness of local water supply. *Lancet*, i, pp. 988-92.

DHSS (1974). *Present day practice in infant feeding.* Department of Health and Social Security Report, London.

DHSS (1978). *Eating for health.* Department of Health and Social Security Report. HMSO, London.

DHSS (1981). *Artificial feeds for the young infant.* Department of Health and Social Security Report. HMSO, London.

Dickie, N. H. and Bender, A. H. (1982). Breakfast and performance in school children. *British Journal of Nutrition* **20**, pp. 483.

Douglas, J. W. B. and Waller, R. E. (1966). Air pollution and respiratory infection in children. *British Journal of Preventive and Social Medicine* **20**, pp. 1–8.

Gardner, M. J., Crawford, M. D., and Morris, J. N. (1969). Pattern of mortality in middle and early old age in the county boroughs of England and Wales. *British Journal of Preventative and Social Medicine* **23**, pp. 133–40.

Golding, J. (1984). Britain's national cohort studies. In *Progress in child health Volume 1* (ed. J. A. Macfarlane), Churchill Livingstone, Edinburgh.

Golding, J. (1986). Child health and the environment. *British Medical Bulletin* **42**(2), pp. 204–11.

Gould, M. S. and Shaffer, D. (1986). The impact of suicide in television movies: evidence of imitation. *New England Journal of Medicine* **315**, pp. 690–4.

Gardner, M. J., Crawford, M. D., and Morris, J. N. (1969). Pattern of mortality in middle and early old age in the county boroughs of England and Wales. *British Journal of Preventive and Social Medicine* **23**, pp. 133–40.

Graham, P. (1979) Epidemiological studies. In *Phychological Disorders of Childhood, 2nd edition* (eds H. C. Quay and J. Werry) pp. 185–209. Wiley, New York.

Jackson, R. H. and Gaffin, J. (1983). The Childhood Accident Prevention Trust. *Archives of Disease in Childhood* **58**, pp. 1031–3.

Martin, J. and Monk, J. (1982) *Infant Feeding 1980*, Office of Population Censuses and Surveys, London.

Miller, F., Court, S. D. M., Knox, E. R., and Brandon, S. (1974). *The school years in Newcastle-upon-Tyne 1955–62*. Oxford University Press, Oxford.

Moore, M. R., Goldberg, A., Morton Fyfe, W., and Richards, W. N. (1981). Maternal lead levels after alterations to water supply. *Lancet* **ii**, pp. 203–4.

Oppe, T. E. (1980). Nutritional strategy—the British scene. In *Topics in paediatrics* (ed. B. A. Wharton), Pitman Medical, London.

Osborn, A. F., Butler, N. R., and Morris, A. C. (1985). *The social life of Britain's five year olds*. Churchill Livingstone, Edinburgh.

Phillips, D. P. and Carstensen, L. L. (1986). Clustering of teenage suicides after television news stories about suicide. *New England Journal of Medicine* **315**, pp. 685–9.

Rutter, M. (1981). *Maternal deprivation reassessed*. Penguin Books, Harmondsworth, Middx.

Rutter, M. (1987a) Continuities and discontinuities from infancy. In *Handbook of Infant Development, 2nd edition* (ed. J. Osofsky) pp. 1256–96. Wiley, New York.

Rutter, M. (1987*b*) Parental mental disorder as a psychiatric risk factor.In *American Psychiatric Association's Annual Review vol 6* (eds R. E. Hales and A. J. Frances) pp. 647–63. Washington, D.C. American Psychiatric Press Inc.

Rutter, M., Yule, B., Morton, J., and Bagley, C. (1975). Attainment and adjustment in two geographical areas: 3. Some factors accounting for area differences. *British Journal of Psychiatry* **126**, pp. 520–33.

Spiers, P. S., Wright, S. G., and Siegel, D. G. (1974). Infant mortality and water hardness in the United States. *Pediatrics* **54**(3), pp. 317–19.

Werner, E. E. (1983), *Kith, kin and hired hands: a cross-cultural view of alternative caregivers for children*. University Park Press, Baltimore, MD.

Zigler, E. F. and Gordon, E. W. (eds.) (1982). *Day care: scientific and social policy issues*. Auburn House, Boston, MA.

A fuller list of references may be obtained from Dr Jean Golding.

6

Health services for children and their relationship to the educational and social services

AIDAN MACFARLANE and ROSS MITCHELL

Introduction

The care of children is primarily the responsibility of their parents, or those acting as their parents. Statutory and voluntary services are intended to help parents in their task. Many parents meet a large proportion of their children's requirements, others satisfy them only partially, and a few hardly at all. Every child has some needs which are beyond the capacity of the parents to meet unaided, while some children have special needs over and above these. Services must therefore be flexible and responsive to a wide range of individual demand.

Parents are responsible for maintaining their children's health, for recognizing illness, and for seeking help from the medical services available. In addition children benefit from the wider public health measures concerned with sanitation, the supply of safe food, and the eradication of disease, which safeguard the health and well-being of the population as a whole. The state of a child's health has implications for education, because a child who is unwell or has some form of continuing disability cannot benefit fully from educational opportunities. Scholastic education is provided for all children by the State but the important contribution made by parents to general education and preparation for living must not be undervalued.

When socio-economic circumstances are not conducive to good child-rearing, the health of children is liable to be adversely affected. There is a close relationship between child health and social conditions. The social needs of children are met by a wide range of provisions—for safety and protection, law and order, play and recreation, and social amenities in general: only when these facilities are insufficient or inappropriate is it necessary for the social service departments to take specific action.

The State has a duty to ensure that all children are properly cared for. Parents do not have exclusive proprietorial authority over their children and recognition of this has been accelerated by increasing realization of the extent of child abuse and neglect by a small minority of parents. Children have rights of their own which must be respected and protected. These rights are enshrined in the Declaration of the Rights of the Child made by the General Assembly of the United Nations in 1959.

Children's needs vary considerably at different ages. The infant requires almost complete care, including feeding, warmth, cleanliness, and protection from harm. As he grows, he can express his own wants to an increasing extent, although the young child continues to need guidance on such matters as safety and hygiene. With greater independence and the start of formal education come more opportunities for self-expression, risk-taking attuned to experience, and social intercourse with peers and other members of his community. An adolescent can largely create these opportunities for himself but in addition requires advice on social and sexual behaviour and counselling about future career and other aspects of adult life. At all ages children need care in illness and affection and companionship best supplied by loving parents and a warm accepting home

In Britain until the last century the services required to meet these manifold needs were non-existent or fragmentary but they gradually evolved from 1870 onwards to attain their maximum development about 1970. Since then financial stringency and changes in political philosophy have resulted in a slowing-down in the development of the child health services and have placed a greater emphasis on parental responsibility. While this has made little difference to families with adequate resources, it bears heavily on the increasing number of parents who are unable to meet the basic requirements of their children because of poverty and unemployment, social deprivation, disintegration of family life, or, in some cases, a disinclination to acknowledge their responsibilities.

Statutory services, whether provided by central government or local authority, tend to develop gradually in response to the recognition of deficiencies, public demand, and political pressures. Once established, such services are slow to change, because the combined effect of bureaucratic inertia, vested interests, and suspicion of anything unfamiliar is to maintain the status quo. Only when provision becomes manifestly inadequate or major abuse is exposed may legislation be introduced to effect improvement. The strength of voluntary effort is that private agencies can act as quickly as need is perceived, can alter direction rapidly, and are not so bound by rigid conditions and restrictions. All too often, however, rivalry between agencies in the same field and complacent acceptance of what has been achieved prevent the adaptation at which the voluntary sector should excel.

There is thus considerable resistance to innovation in all services. Often it is a major cataclysm, such as war and its aftermath, which seems to create conditions conducive to substantial change. Thus the Children's Charter of 1908 closely followed the events of the Boer War and there were important advances in child health care after the First World War with the creation of the maternity and child welfare services largely as we know them today. In the years following the Second World War, the National Health Service (NHS) was introduced, and local authority children's departments, later incorporated into enlarged social service departments (social work departments in Scotland), were established. In the past four decades, there has been no comparable social upheaval and perhaps this accounts, at least in part, for the difficulties encountered in transforming services to enable them to meet the changing needs of children more effectively. Some of the reasons why more appropriate child health services have been slow to materialize are the complexity of the services themselves and the lack of radical planning and necessary reorganization; the conservatism of the medical profession along with a degree of unwarranted complacency in all sections of society; the 'emotional' weighting given to certain childhood diseases which apportions greater resources to them than are warranted by their frequency; and the paucity of relevant research and peer audit.

Another factor preventing the evolution of better services and the creation of an integrated child health service is that existing staff, fearing loss of employment or new demands to be made on them, have been reluctant to contemplate changes. Over-emphasis on 'who does what' and the status accorded to different kinds of work have tended to obscure the central issue of meeting children's needs and have impeded the implementation of new ideas. Inertia has been accentuated by lack of enthusiasm amongst civil servants and administrators for necessary changes involving extra work and expense at a time when staffs are depleted and budgets tight.

These and other constraints should not be allowed to compromise the interests of children and their families. They must be countered by reasoned argument emphasizing the importance of creating children's services specifically designed to meet new needs effectively and efficiently, rather than half-heartedly tinkering with services that have become inappropriate to modern requirements. In this chapter we outline the existing health services for children, discuss their relationship with the educational and social services, indicate their weaknesses, and suggest how they should be reconstructed.

Children's services in the 1980s

Health services

Meeting health needs One aim of the health services is to aid parents as the primary protectors and managers of their child's health. Only in certain circumstances should the service itself take on this role. One of these is childbirth, for in this country almost all pregnancies and deliveries are supervised by the obstetric services and all the resulting new-born infants receive some care from health service staff. A minority of new-born infants will require special measures of investigation or treatment. Following delivery, about one-third of mothers will be visited at home by health visitors during the first six months of the child's life and over three-quarters of the children will be taken to child health clinics. Children who manifest symptoms attributed to illness will usually be cared for by their parents without reference to or contact with the medical services, since the great majority of such episodes are minor disturbances. When the general practitioner is consulted, only 3 per cent of these consultations will result in referral to hospital. None the less, one in every four children is admitted to hospital at some time during the first five years.

In the UK, health services are largely provided by the NHS, intended from its start in 1948 to provide comprehensive health care for the whole family. During its first two decades the maintenance of child health was shared between the NHS and local authorities operating separately. These functions were merged statutorily (if not very effectively functionally) in 1974, when the health services were reorganized. Reviews of the ways in which health care was delivered to children were undertaken in the late 1960s: the findings for Scotland were published in the Brotherston Report (1973) and for England and Wales in the Court Report (1976). Both reports criticized the separation between primary health care, hospital services, and services in the community; deplored the inadequacy of cooperation between the different sectors and the consequent duplication and discontinuity of services; and recommended that children's services should be more clearly identified by integrating the general practice, hospital, and community components into a single child health service within the NHS. Such a coalescence would have promoted efficacy and efficiency and allowed better evaluation and quality control. However, despite much discussion and expressions of intent, the recommendations of these reports have not been implemented, except in a few minor respects, and the service remains fragmented. Effectively, there are three main parts. General practitioners provide the bulk of treatment and some of the preventive care (primary care); doctors in the community child health clinics and school clinics (clinical medical officers) are responsible for much of the preventive care and school health work; and consultants in hospitals and clinics undertake the more specialized forms of care (secondary care), including the management of complex forms of health relating to education.

This tripartite structure, with child care interspersed amongst services for the whole population, has a number of disadvantages financial and otherwise, not least that communication between the different parts is not always as good as it should be. While the shortcomings imposed by this uneconomic tripartite structure might have been made good in more expansive and affluent times, the financial stringency imposed on the NHS since the late 1970s has meant the increasing diversion of funds to meet the needs of the aged and the burgeoning demands of ever more costly technological medicine. In this competitive climate, the needs of children have been accorded a lower priority and the necessary move towards greater integration of child health services, as envisaged by the Court and Brotherston Committees, has been checked. Nevertheless, the Court and Brotherston Reports and the resultant greater awareness of the deficiencies of child health care in Britain have led to closer analysis of professional work, more appropriate medical education, and a consequent trend towards better paediatric care by family doctors.

In theory every child in the country receives adequate primary health care but the reality is that there are children, especially in large housing estates, inner city areas of deprivation, and poorly served rural areas, whose health is not properly supervised. In these circumstances, when lock-up surgeries, deputizing services, and hospital accident and emergency departments replace the personal family doctor, the service provided is less than satisfactory, whilst the concomitants of deprivation—poverty, helplessness, and apathy—militate against families using such services as are available.

Responsibility for the planning of child health services lies ultimately with the regional and district health authorities. Each district in England and Wales has a Joint Care Planning Team (JCPT) (Fig. 6.1) to identify and bridge gaps in provision between health, social, educational, and housing services, where these relate to community care. The activities of the JCPT are aimed specifically at children and families with special needs, as well as the mentally ill or handicapped, the elderly, and the younger physically handicapped people. A special fund, independent of the normal health and social service budgets, finances projects set up by the JCPT, money being allocated by the Department of Health and Social Security to regional authorities, which then distribute it to districts. Projects recommended by the JCPT must be approved by a Joint Consultative Committee (JCC) (Fig. 6.1) with members from the health and social service authorities, the district or borough councils, and voluntary organizations. The JCC then puts forward proposals which have to be agreed independently by the health and social service authorities. Projects financed in this way may or may not have long-term revenue consequences. In the former case, funding is usually for three years, thereafter tapering off during a further five years. One or other of the authorities concerned agrees to take over the longer term costs after JCPT funding has ceased. These planning responsibilities are shown in Fig. 6.1. An average health authority district might be allocated between £500 000 and £100 000 per annum for these special projects.

The interrelationship of the principal services for children is shown in Fig. 6.2.

Preventive health services The paradox of prevention is that the better it works the less conscious people are that it is working and

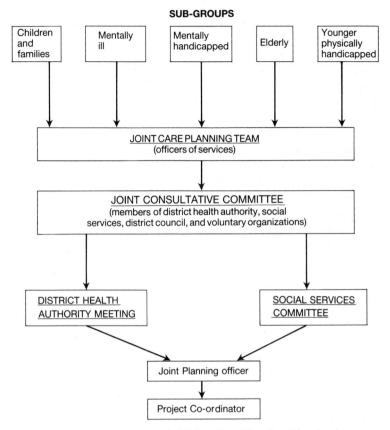

Fig. 6.1. Structure of Joint Care Planning Team.

so its value is likely to be underrated. Preventive measures may be considered at three levels—primary, secondary, and tertiary.

Primary prevention refers to the prevention of a disease from occurring in the first place. Probably the single most effective measure is to provide the best possible socio-economic environment, for virtually all disease is more common when children are brought up in adverse social conditions, whether these be in terms of poverty, poor housing, parental unemployment, neglect, or a combination of such factors. Other primary preventive measures leading to improved child health include genetic counselling of parents before conception; prevention of unwanted pregnancies by family planning; immunization against tuberculosis, diphtheria,

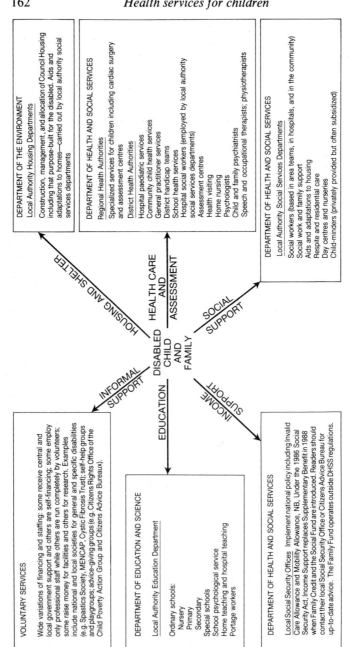

Fig. 6.2. Principal services for disabled children showing responsibilities and interrelationships. The provisions outlined are those for England, and may differ in Scotland, Wales, and Northern Ireland. Not all the services listed will be available in every health authority or local district, since resources, policies, and practices vary. (Kindly prepared by Mrs Jean Gaffin, Executive Secretary, British Paediatric Association.)

tetanus, whooping cough, poliomyelitis, and measles; fostering or adoption of children neglected or abandoned by their parents; the fluoridation of water and toothpaste in the prevention of dental caries; health education of parents, children, and the general public.

Secondary prevention means that although a disease has occurred its long-term effects are prevented; e.g. when the hip joint of the new-born infant is found to be dislocated and the condition is effectively treated before damage to the hip ensues, or when otitis media (infection of the middle ear) is treated early so that deafness is prevented. Other secondary preventable conditions recognizable at birth include phenylketonuria, a metabolic disease occurring in one in 10 000 infants which, if not corrected by dietary means, will lead to mental retardation, and hypothyroidism (affecting about one in 3500) which, if not treated early, will result in progressive developmental delay. Other examples are one type of sensorineural deafness (about one per 1000) which can be helped by use of a hearing aid in the first year of life, and strabismus (squint) which can cause blindness in the squinting eye if not detected and treated early. In genetic terms secondary prevention is often applied to the termination of pregnancy where a grossly abnormal fetus has been diagnosed during the early weeks.

Tertiary prevention is where difficulties associated with a handicapping disorder are identified and dealt with before they can cause further handicap; e.g. joint contractures in cerebral palsy or incipient behaviour disturbances in mentally handicapped children. Such identification is usually made when a coordinated multiprofessional assessment involving specialists such as the paediatrician, psychologist, orthopaedic surgeon, geneticist, physiotherapist, occupational therapist, speech therapist, audiologist, orthoptist, and possibly others is undertaken within a short space of time. An example of tertiary prevention is the diagnosis of visual and hearing disorders in children with Down's syndrome. They have a relatively high incidence of these abnormalities, and correction with glasses and hearing aids achieves a better quality of life.

General preventive measures are those intended to improve the environment. Preventive measures constitute an important and growing function of the child health services and have greatly increased the demand on the community health services. New techniques of diagnosis and treatment, with their implications for secondary and tertiary prevention, call for additional resources of staff and equipment both in hospitals and in the community. As examples, selective abortion of fetuses with major malformations, while it will reduce the incidence of children with congenital abnormalities, imposes a further work-load on laboratory and obstetric services. Provision of expensive intensive care facilities for new-born infants requires expansion to rectify its present deficiencies. Although primarily therapeutic, perinatal care has important preventive implications, since monitoring the condition of the fetus and new-born infant and correcting deviations from normal help to prevent complications of birth and immaturity.

Child health surveillance   Health surveillance for the pre-school child is mainly undertaken at child health clinics and for the schoolchild by the school health service. Surveillance includes monitoring growth and development, implementing a programme of preventive measures, and giving advice and support to parents. A key person in pre-school health surveillance is the health visitor, a highly trained nurse who works both in the clinic and in the child's home. The doctor's role is usually met by clinical medical officers but increasingly general practitioners are arranging their own clinics for the children in their practices.

In the child health clinic, children are immunized against a range of communicable diseases and screened for various abnormalities, such as congenital dislocation of the hip, undescended testes, visual and hearing defects, and disorders of growth. At appropriate intervals the general developmental progress of the child is assessed. While serious deviations from the normal pattern will be recognized, the efficiency of developmental screening tests is not high, because a relatively large number of children who fail them turn out to be normal and some who pass the tests do have developmental problems. The value of assessing development lies mainly in the examination of the child in the presence of the parents, who can observe and discuss their child's performance. Routine testing is also useful for teaching professional staff about the range of normal development, so that they become expert at determining whether an apparent deviation from normal warrants reassurance or referral for further attention.

Well over 50 per cent of parents attend child health clinics in order to obtain advice and reassurance. In one study (Sefi and

Macfarlane 1985) of 1000 visits by mothers to clinics, 30 per cent thought that meeting other mothers and getting their advice was helpful, 40 per cent valued counselling and reassurance from the doctor, and 50 per cent found the advice of the health visitor to be of benefit.

The number of child health clinics in each health district in relation to the pre-school population varies greatly, some districts having four times as many clinics per head of the under-five-years-old population as the least well-provided districts. There appears to be no good reason why this should be so: it is presumably due to historical factors in the way the child health services have been established in each district. The need for child health clinics divorced from general practice should gradually diminish in those areas where increasing numbers of general practitioners undertake surveillance of the children in their own practices.

One of the main purposes of health surveillance is to detect abnormalities which require treatment or more detailed study. It is sometimes the first stage in a process which may involve further evaluation and investigation, specialized treatment, and continuing management, perhaps for many years. Of particular importance is the identification at an early stage of those children who may later have special educational needs and the notification of such children to the educational authorities. More research is needed to determine how successful are surveillance programmes in achieving this aim.

Primary health care An important part of the primary care of children is the diagnosis of disease and trauma, the investigation of these, the provision of such treatment as is required, and the management of the situation created by the illness or injury. Primary health care in the UK is carried out by a large number of people in addition to parents and children themselves, notably by general practitioners, clinical medical officers in child health clinics, audiologists, orthoptists and ophthalmologists, dentists, and teachers. Although all these and others have important parts to play in primary care, in common parlance the 'primary health care team' refers to the general practitioner, staff directly employed by the practice, and the health visitors working with the practice, who are employed by the district health authority.

About one-third of the total work-load in general practice is concerned with children under the age of 15 years, the proportion varying in different practices. Health visitors, however, spend a large part of their time, perhaps as much as 75 per cent or more, with children. An important role of both general practitioner and health visitor is the coordination of all the child care services, ensuring that they interact and that staff liaise to the benefit of the child and the family.

Ninety per cent of all children less than five years old are taken to see the family doctor each year. Of such consultations, 90 per cent will be for relatively minor, self-limiting illness, with only 3 per cent ending in referral to hospital. In one representative practice, the pattern of illness seen in children up to 14 years of age, in terms of consultations each year per 1000 children, was as shown in Table 6.1. For pre-school children, the referral rates to hospital from this general practice were as shown in Table 6.2.

About 6 per cent of pre-school children will be seen by their family doctor because of long-term disability. In the practice referred to, the children on the 'handicap register' are shown in Table 6.3.

How frequently do general practitioners see congenital malformations in children? Taking the average practice of 2500 patients, a doctor will encounter new cases at the frequency rates shown in Table 6.4.

Hitherto the primary care of children has usually been based on responding to calls initiated by parents when their child is ill or they believe something is wrong. However, increasing numbers of general practitioners are undertaking regular developmental testing as part of health surveillance, the children being seen with their parents at consultations initiated by the doctor himself. These not only help to detect abnormalities at an early stage but also provide a valuable opportunity for the doctor to discuss with the parents any problems or anxieties they may have about their child.

Specialist health care Better training and facilities in general practice enable family doctors to care for some children who would formerly have been sent to hospital. This might have been expected to diminish the number of hospital admissions of children but paradoxically the numbers have been increasing, despite the fall in the child population, because childhood disorders are now recognized and referred to hospital at an earlier stage and parents know and expect more of the services. Moreover, modern in-

Table 6.1

Pattern of illness seen in two age groups in one representative practice.

	No. consultations/year/1000 children	
Disease or symptom	0−4 years	5−14 years
Respiratory disease	1009	521
Upper respiratory tract infection	470	152
Tonsillitis	213	186
Bronchitis	183	73
Otitis media	168	83
Catarrh	48	22
Ill-defined symptoms	343	168
Cough	113	49
Vomiting/diarrhoea	112	31
Infective	209	160
Measles/rubella/chicken-pox	84	51

Table 6.2

Referral rates from general practice to hospital for pre-school children (0−4 years old) in one representative practice.

Annual (general practice) consultations (0−4 years old)	725
Referrals to hospital out-patient departments	8
Referrals for in-patient care	2
Referrals for other investigations	8
Total referrals as percentage of annual consultations	2.4

vestigation and treatment are often complex, requiring careful monitoring, and so hospital supervision may be necessary for longer periods of time. The net result is that, while the duration of stay in hospital has been substantially reduced, the number of children attending out-patient departments and admitted to hospital has grown.

With the advance of medical knowledge and skill, the hospital care of children has become increasingly specialized. It therefore becomes all the more important to consider every aspect of the child's life in relation to any illness or injury suffered as well as the impact on the family. An episode of illness can be an upsetting

Table 6.3

Number of pre-school children (0−4 years old) with various disabilities seen in one representative practice.

Total number of pre-school children	1500
Behaviour disorders	28
Asthma	24
Neurological disorders	9
Skeletal disorders	6
Metabolic disorders	5
Mental subnormality	4
Cardiovascular disorders	2
Sensory disorders	4
Total number of disabilities (and as a percentage of total number of children)	82 (5.4)

Table 6.4

Frequency rates of encounter of congenital malformations in children in a representative practice of 2500 patients.

Malformation	Seen once in every
Congenital malformation of the heart	5 years
Pyloric stenosis	7 years
Talipes (club foot)	7 years
Spina bifida	7 years
Down's syndrome	10 years
Cleft palate	20 years
Congenital dislocation of the hip	20 years
Bifid penis	2000 years

experience, especially for a young child, and if it is accompanied by separation from the family and by fear and/or pain the emotional disturbance may be severe and its effects long lasting. Children should not therefore be admitted to hospital unless absolutely necessary and then one or other of the parents should stay with their child as much as possible. Every child who requires admission should be in a children's unit with staff trained and experienced in the care of children and equipment specifically intended for paediatric use. General hospital staff caring for patients of all ages cannot be expected to have sufficient understanding of child development to minimize emotional disturbance nor have they the continuing experience necessary to care for infants and small children in an expert and sensitive way.

Even experienced paediatric staff cannot use their skills effectively if their equipment is designed for adults and unsuitable for children. Given the specialization, knowledge, understanding, and experience to be found in a large hospital unit specifically for children, with equipment expressly intended for paediatric use, all the investigative and therapeutic resources of modern medicine should be available to every child who needs them. This implies liaison with services for adults and clearly all facilities cannot be provided in every hospital. There is thus a need for regional and national planning of specialized services for children, often limiting them to certain centres so that it is then necessary to send or transfer some children to a distant hospital to obtain the best treatment. Parents generally accept the need for this, if the reason is explained, though it creates problems for them in trying to maintain close links with their child in hospital. Difficulties can be countered by arranging accommodation for parents in or near the hospital and by providing for the cost of their travel as of right.

The need to admit children to hospital is reduced if there are good day-care facilities, and increasing numbers of hospitals have purpose-built day units for children. Here again, things are made easier for parents if there is family accommodation close to the hospital, especially if day care is likely to extend to several days. Admission may also be avoided in many instances when there is a well-equipped out-patient department supported by the full diagnostic and therapeutic resources of the hospital (Plate VIII). Whenever possible, such clinics should be exclusively for children's use and designed and decorated expressly for them. While out-patient consultations are best conducted under such optimal conditions, the concentration of in-patient care in centralized children's units large enough to meet the highest standards implies the need to provide dispersed paediatric out-patient expertise in clinics distant from the main hospital. Much can be achieved in an out-patient consultation by an experienced paediatrician with only minimal facilities, though inevitably some children will have to be seen at the paediatric department.

Hospital care for infants and children is provided by a range of consultants and specialists, supported by a great variety of other hospital staff. All doctors caring for children should have training in paediatrics. In an age of increasing specialization in individual organs or systems of the body, it is important that some consultants maintain a high level of expertise in general aspects of child life and health, growth and development, and the diseases which affect infants and children. Such general paediatricians collaborate closely with family doctors and provide secondary care for the majority of children who require medical treatment in hospital. A proportion of ill children need the particular skill of a paediatric system specialist, such as a paediatric cardiologist or neurologist, or sometimes of a system specialist with experience of a particular disease in patients of all ages, who then works in consultation with a general paediatrician.

Most new-born infants are under the supervision of a general paediatrician but in large maternity units providing intensive neonatal care, including such care for infants referred from other maternity units, there are usually paediatricians who specialize in this field. At the other end of the age range, adolescence is a period of transition, after which children with continuing disease or disability pass from the care of the paediatrician to the appropriate specialist for adults. This transfer of responsibility must be carefully arranged in consultation with the family doctor to avoid detrimental loss of continuity. There is a need for more and more varied facilities for adolescents, including arrangements for paediatricians, general physicians, and psychiatrists to work together in this field.

In the largest centres, there are general and orthopaedic surgeons, otolaryngologists (ear, nose, and throat consultants), ophthalmologists (consultants in diseases of the eye), and others who confine their practice to children, but in most hospitals these specialists see patients of all ages. When dealing with children they often work in collaboration with a paediatrician who advises on growth and development, nutrition, and other aspects of child health in relation to the child's particular disorder. Child psychiatrists also work closely with paediatricians but their approach is rather different, for they are children's specialists who, though child-centred, necessarily work also with adult patients in the context of family psychiatry.

Outside the hospital, secondary health care is provided by a large number of professionals, including consultant paediatricians working both in and out of hospital. Many of these have particular interest in continuing disabilities, such as cerebral palsy or language and learning disorders, while others specialize in chronic diseases such as diabetes, asthma, or cystic fibrosis. Various community health doctors and others now participate in hospital-based services, so that the divisions between hospital and community are disappearing and the hospital is increasingly viewed as one resource, albeit an important one, in an integrated pattern of health care for the whole child population. The professional staff of this child health service include doctors and nurses, physiotherapists, occupational therapists and speech therapists, psychologists, orthoptists, dentists, and many others. They work in hospitals, schools, and clinics, in centres for the assessment and management of handicapped children, and as members of child development teams and district handicap teams. They collaborate closely with teachers and social workers, especially concerning children with special needs, estimated variously at 10 to 20 per cent of the child population. Almost all these children spend most of their time at home or in school, although they make frequent visits to hospital clinics, and both they and their parents need continuing support from health, educational, and social services.

The coordination of the secondary care services lies mainly with consultant paediatricians, many of whom have a special community interest, and senior clinical medical officers working with the health visitors, school nurses, and other professional staff and cooperating with the general practitioners and clinical medical officers who provide primary care. Community medicine specialists have an important role in planning child health services to take account of epidemiological, social, and geographical factors. The task of integrating services, particularly those for children with special needs, calls for ever more complex management and equipment and for closer communication with hospital staff and the educational and social services.

Health in relation to educational services

Pre-school children   Children in the UK usually start school at the age of five years but there is a large and growing demand for education in the pre-school years. General education for living is largely the responsibility of parents but they may be helped in this task by professional workers skilled in developing the abilities of young children, and through play providing an informal learning process which is an essential part of the child's whole education. Many children have some form of pre-school group activity, at playgroup, day nursery, or nursery school, but there is increasing pressure to make these facilities more widely available, especially as it is now clear that pre-school experience affords significant benefits to children in their subsequent education.

Early education is particularly important for children with disabilities. Their special needs make a longer period of formal learning essential if they are to fulfil their potential. The majority of these children should attend the same groups and nursery schools as children who have no special needs, for such integration is to their advantage. The minority who are unable for one reason or another to attend early group education of this type should be visited by peripatetic teachers in their homes. Health authorities which are conscious of the close links between health and education at this age arrange medical supervision of centres for pre-school education and encourage liaison with peripatetic teachers.

The Education Act (1981) makes it mandatory for the health services to try to identify children who have, or may in the future have, special educational needs. In some cases a child's disability will be recognized at birth, e.g. Down's syndrome, or in early infancy, e.g. many forms of cerebral palsy. Sometimes slow development will alert parents or the health visitor to the possibility that something is wrong, or screening tests at the child health clinic may reveal a disability. In yet other instances a difficulty requiring special educational measures will not be recognized until after school entry, e.g. some forms of learning disorder. If parents suspect a disability they should seek the advice of their family doctor, who will usually arrange for the child to be seen by a paediatrician. If appropriate the paediatrician will coordinate further specialist investigation as the start of a planned programme to meet the child's future needs.

If a child is under the age of two years when special needs are identified the parents have the option of deciding whether or not to have a multiprofessional assessment of their child's probable strengths and weaknesses; over the age of two, the health authority has a statutory obligation to inform the education authority of any child having special educational needs. The education authority may then decide (1) to have a multiprofessional assessment of the child; (2) subsequently to arrange for a statement of that child's educational needs; and (3) what the content of that statement should be. In all three instances, the parents can appeal against the decision of the education authority.

School health   The primary objectives of the school health service in relation to the education of children and support for the schools, as stated for the London Education Authority (Court Report 1976), are as follows: (1) to promote the understanding and practice of child health and paediatrics in relation to the process of learning; (2) to provide a continuing service of health surveillance and medical protection throughout the years of childhood and adolescence; (3) to recognize and ensure the proper management of what may broadly be described as medical, surgical, and neurodevelopmental disorders in so far as they may influence, directly or indirectly, the child's learning and social development, particularly at school but also at home; (4) to ensure that parents and teachers are aware of the presence of such disorders and of their significance for the child's education and care; (5) to give advice and service to the education authority as required in the 1981 Education Act and the 1974 NHS Act.

The professional background to the school health service is the practice of educational medicine, defined as the study and practice of child health and paediatrics in relation to the processes of learning.

It requires an understanding of child development, the educational environment, the child's response to schooling, the disorders which interfere with a child's capacity to learn, and the special needs of the handicapped. Its practitioners need to work co-operatively with the teachers, psychologists and others who may be involved with the child and to understand the influences of family and social environment (Court Report 1976).

Clearly this is a specialist field which must be practised within the schools themselves; hence every school should have its own designated school doctor who has been appropriately trained in educational medicine. Most state schools do have such a school doctor, who may be a general practitioner with sessions in the school or, more commonly, a doctor working in the community child health services. All school children should of course have their own family doctor but it is not feasible for every family doctor to supervise the school progress of his own patients, so there must be a single doctor relating to each school who will cooperate with the family doctors in providing total primary care.

At more specialized levels, especially those relating to children with special needs, educational medicine is practised by consultant paediatricians with an interest in this field and by senior clinical medical officers. Such doctors are trained and experienced in the recognition and assessment of disorders causing learning difficulties and in cooperating with teachers in the management of these problems. They consult in ordinary schools as well as working in special schools, assessment centres, and other clinics.

A key member of the school health team is the specially trained school nurse, who shares responsibility with the school doctor, the two collaborating very closely together. The school nurse spends most of her time in the school, acquires an intimate knowledge of the children and their parents and teachers, and plays a major part in health education, the administration of medicines during school hours and their safe-keeping, and the maintenance and confidential handling of school health records.

Health education   Many of the disorders that afflict modern society are related to patterns of personal behaviour, so that attempts to establish a healthy life-style should begin early, by health education and health promotion in the schools. While much informal shaping of attitudes goes on in the classroom, health education should be a subject for serious study in the school curriculum. This is a joint responsibility of health and educational authorities but there are no clear national guidelines about what should be included, and the head-teacher, school doctor, and school nurse have to decide amongst themselves the content and presentation of health education in their school.

Many of the problems of health promotion in schools today concern the taking of drugs such as alcohol, tobacco, marijuana, and other 'harder' kinds. A survey (Macfarlane) of 643 fourteen-year-old children in one health district showed that, although 98 per cent of the children thought that smoking would harm their health, 21 per cent still smoked. Nearly all (95 per cent) had had an alcoholic drink at some time, 43 per cent within the last week, and 30 per cent drank regularly every week. Of those children who smoked, 52 per cent drank at least once a week, 19 per cent had sniffed glue, and 29 per cent had tried other drugs. Of the non-smokers, 24 per cent drank at least once a week, only 2 per cent had sniffed glue, and 4 per cent had tried other drugs. The respective roles of educational and health services in seeking to prevent drug abuse are not clear but the objectives are likely to be achieved most effectively by joint action between the two services.

Increasing numbers of handicapped children are being integrated into ordinary schools, rather than segregated in special schools, as the benefits of more realistic competition are appreciated and the rights of all children to participate as fully as possible in the life of their community are acknowledged. For integration to succeed, adequate resources to meet special needs must be provided in all schools and teachers must be made more aware of the problems. The information given to them has to be radically reviewed, with revision of written material and fresh approaches provided by school doctors and nurses. Teachers are not expected to become 'mini doctors' or to undergo long training courses on the management of the handicapped, but do require to have more understanding of, and in some instances a change of attitude towards, children with disabilities. Medical information about the condition and needs of the individual child should be readily available, so that the teacher can appreciate what is being recommended, and why, and can make a more informed contribution to the child's education.

Health in relation to social services

The background Standards of child health are inextricably interwoven with the quality of child and family life, which partly depends on the availability and use of social services. The latter cannot therefore be considered separately from health services, for any reduction in one is likely to result in increased demands on the other. The growth of social services in the UK between 1950 and 1970 might have been expected to result in better health as well as a better quality of life for all children.

Some global criteria of child life and health did improve but a serious gap between the poorest and the most affluent families remained and has widened since 1980. Thus more than one in every eight families in the UK receives social security payments and over one-quarter of all children are living close to or below the margin of poverty. Perinatal mortality is twice as high in the infants of parents in unskilled manual occupations as in those of professional parents, and similar gradients of disadvantage are evident when other measures of health are applied to different occupational groups. These social differences are reflected in the inequalities in child health that were described in the Black Report (DHSS 1980). They are accentuated by unemployment, which imposes strains on family life in addition to those of poverty. It is against this background that the social services for children must be considered.

Statutory and voluntary services   In years gone by, a family in difficulties relied largely on relatives and friends for help but gradually a system of state support evolved, amplified by private philanthropy. Local authority social services, which grew rapidly between 1950 and 1970, were reorganized in 1968 with the idea of providing a single door for help and advice. On balance the composite social service department (social work department in Scotland) has worked well, reducing gaps in service and duplication of effort, but has the disadvantage that a family unsuccessful in obtaining assistance from the social service department has no other portal of entry, for the 'safety net' of multiple or specialist points of contact has been lost. In these circumstances specialist voluntary agencies have flourished, often with the encouragement of local authority departments, which may not have the resources to meet particular need themselves. Thus, for example, a substantial proportion of residential accommodation for children is provided by voluntary bodies, the cost being met in part by local authorities, which have a statutory duty to make suitable provision.

Every person can and should have a family doctor and there is generally no hesitation in using the health services. The same cannot be said of the social services, although their hope is that ultimately everyone will welcome the idea of the personal social worker comparable with the general medical practitioner. At present, however, families tend to call on social workers only when the need is pressing, and the social service departments deal largely with children who are disadvantaged socially and educationally. While many families do use the services as of right, recourse to a social worker still carries a stigma for some people and contact may therefore be made only with reluctance. In such families, the health visitor may be accepted more readily, and accordingly it is essential for health and social services to cooperate in close harmony, so that appropriate help can be provided where it is needed.

The interdependence of health and social circumstances and the complexity of the interaction between them mean that virtually all social support has some implication for health. The most immediate and direct way in which the social services complement the child health services is by cooperation between a social worker and the primary health care team in the interests of a particular child. This may entail improving the home environment by advice and/or material help, assisting the family to obtain full benefit from the health measures recommended, or arranging for the care and protection of children in need because of family disruption or parental abuse. Less directly, the efforts of the social services to improve living standards and their work in connection with legislative aspects of child life have had general effects in improving child health.

A high proportion of underprivileged families are in contact with social service departments, whereas the more affluent often feel self-sufficient and do not seek help. Paradoxically, less deprived parents tend to be more articulate and competent at seeking out and benefiting from the services, while families living at or near the margin of poverty may not make effective use of the resources that are available. Some of their difficulty may relate to the size, standing, and powers of local authorities, and smaller, less official, voluntary agencies may be able to establish a better relationship with these families.

The wide range of attitudes and needs among clients means that every social agency, whether statutory or voluntary, has to be sensitive to varying requirements and prepared to adapt to circumstances, so that families receive support as effectively as possible. This is especially important where there are young children, whose requirements may not always be recognized or met by their caretakers. Special attention needs to be directed at unsupported parents, who usually have difficulties over and above those of others in the same material situation.

With so many calls for help and requirements for social support, demand can never be fully met, for it is almost infinite. With limited government funding and voluntary donation, an element of selection is unavoidable. At present this is often opportunistic, determined by the most immediate pressures. One of the major tasks for the social services in the future is to establish priorities on the basis of agreed principles, though voluntary bodies will always wish to direct their efforts towards particular aims of their own choosing.

Fostering and adoption   Nowhere is the need for close cooperation between health and social services more evident than in the practice of fostering and adoption. In this country the nuclear family of parents and their children is held up as the ideal to be achieved if possible or to be imitated if not. It may be supported and strengthened by a network of close relatives but modern urban life and greater social mobility tend increasingly to isolate the nuclear family and throw it on its own resources, subjecting it to strains which may be too great for young parents. When a family unit is disrupted by marital strife or broken by death or divorce, it may be in the best interest of the children for new arrangements to be made for their care. Whether these should be an alternative form of family life or absorption into a larger community will depend on the particular circumstances: often a substitute family will be the best solution but in some situations a child may thrive better in a different kind of environment.

Fostering is the practice of placing a child in another family under supervision, usually for a finite period, which may be short or long term. Most social service departments have difficulty in finding sufficient suitable foster parents, especially as many of the children they seek to place have emotional and personality problems as the result of their past experiences of broken homes, parental disharmony, separation, and the like.

Adoption is a more permanent placement whereby the adoptive parents, after an obligatory trial period, are given full responsibility for the child as a member of their family, with all that that implies. While this may provide many of the elements of a natural family relationship, such as warm affection and continuity of care, it cannot be an exact replica. The pattern of adoption has changed radically in this country following a fall in the number of unwanted illegitimate children. This occurred partly because of the wide use of oral contraceptives and the greater ease of obtaining termination of pregnancy and partly because it has become more acceptable for an unmarried mother to keep her child and to receive encouragement and help to do so. Thus there are usually waiting lists of people anxious to adopt a child but fewer willing to accept a child with a disability or one of different ethnic origin.

As the supply of children for adoption has fallen, the laws and procedures governing the process have been tightened up, with greater awareness of the disastrous consequences of ill-conceived arrangements in past years, when a child was often placed for adoption on the basis of informal ill-considered agreements between interested parties which resulted in parents unsuitable to adopt being able to do so. Today, registered adoption agencies, which may be social service departments or adoption societies, conduct interviews with prospective parents and arrange for their medical examination and for a medical report on the infant to be adopted. Great care is taken to make placements suitable and to supervise the arrangement before the adoption order is finally granted.

Residential care   When a child in care can neither be fostered nor adopted, or the circumstances are such that these procedures would be inappropriate, the alternative is residence in a children's home or residential school. Formerly this was often the easy solution but, with increasing recognition of the potentially adverse effects of life in a children's home, more effort is now made to place a child in a family and there is less ready recourse to residential care.

In the past, many children's homes were institutional, with children regimented in large groups and dressed uniformly, so that individuality tended to be lost. A few homes may still be like that but better understanding of the needs of children in the past several decades has resulted in the establishment of more intimate homes of a less formal nature and the breaking up of large agglomerations of children in the bigger homes into family-size groups. Residential staff are not the children's parents but they may fulfil some parental roles and a family atmosphere can be achieved in parallel with other forms of care in the same institution. Increasingly, children in residential homes spend days or weekends with relatives or friends outside and the description of a child as being 'in local authority care' is becoming less precise as a label.

Health supervision of children in care is usually undertaken by a local general practitioner or sometimes, in the case of a large home, by a visiting doctor from the community child health service. Those responsible for the children's care must ensure that every child has proper medical and dental attention: children's homes and foster homes have to meet general health requirements and both are inspected at regular intervals.

Until recently, the great majority of residential staff were untrained in parentcraft and had little concept of the needs of disadvantaged children in terms of assessment, independence training, behaviour modification, and so on. No doubt the drab routine of former orphanages was often lightened by the kindness and affection of individual attendants but it must have been difficult to extend this to large numbers of children and especially to the less lovable amongst them. Determined and sustained efforts to recruit and train suitable people have resulted in a substantial improvement in standards but there is a continuing shortage of good residential staff, for relatively few will now undertake this work, with its exacting demands and poor emoluments. Despite the advances, therefore, there is still considerable difficulty in finding suitable placements for children for whom residential care is the only option, especially in areas with a high rate of social deprivation.

Neglect and abuse   The causes and manifestations of child abuse and neglect are considered in Chapter 5. The services required for dealing with these difficult problems must necessarily be comprehensive; encompassing family support and the improvement of the physical environment; attempting to identify and obviate potential danger; supervising families at risk; and coping with the situation when a child has been ill-used. Co-operation and mutual regard between workers from health, social work, legal, and police services are essential and in many areas good working arrangements have been established and ways of proceeding agreed.

All health staff have to be alert to the possibility of abuse when dealing with young children, especially those who have sustained injuries. Vigilance is particularly important in the family doctor's surgery and in the hospital accident and emergency department, because abuse is liable to be overlooked when attending to numbers of patients with varying complaints. When there is the slightest indication of ill-treatment, whether physical, sexual, or emotional, the child should be admitted to hospital forthwith and kept there while further investigations are undertaken. If the parents object or try to take their child away, a 'Place of Safety Order' may be obtained by the social worker concerned. The receiving doctor has to take a full history and make a complete examination of the child, including photographs and X-rays, although he must always bear in mind the possibility of some explanation for his findings other than abuse or neglect. If he concludes that abuse has or may have taken place, a senior doctor, generally a consultant paediatrician, should interview the parents to discuss the findings and their implications. The doctor has a duty to inform the appropriate authorities, usually the social service department or other social agency, and this should be explained to the parents.

Children in trouble   Today there are rather more than 5000 children in penal establishments in England and Wales. Yet there may be little or no distinction between juvenile offenders and children in need of care and protection. Socially unacceptable behaviour often has a basis in ill-health or disability which is not recognized at the time. The health services therefore have an important role to play in the diagnosis of a medical component in delinquency, in drawing the attention of the authorities to this, and in recommending and undertaking suitable management programmes.

A new pattern of dealing with children in trouble started in Scotland with the establishment of the Children's Hearing System following the Kilbrandon Report (1964). At a Children's Hearing, three ordinary citizens, from a panel carefully chosen for the work, talk to the parents and child, having first been given the background facts by an official known as the Reporter. If the parents and child admit the offence, discussion centres around what should be done for the child so that he or she does not get into trouble again. Only if the family denies the charge or if the crime is a very serious one is the case referred to a court of law.

The operation of this system depends on being able to provide for a wide variety of individual needs and hitherto the narrow range of options available has tended to limit the potential value of Children's Hearings. Nevertheless, the experiment has been largely successful and the proceedings, which are intended to be helpful and not punitive, represent a more humane and enlightened approach to these difficult and often complex problems. The system has attracted worldwide interest and it is likely that at least some elements of it will be incorporated into the juvenile justice arrangements in other countries, including England and Wales.

Shortcomings in children's services

Throughout this century there have been intermittent but progressive advances towards better services for children. Major leaps forward initiated by public demand and activated by Acts of Parliament have alternated with faltering steps or periods of standstill as interest waned and stimulus ceased. Today, recognized need, increasing parental expectations, and rapid advances in knowledge and professional expertise mean that demand is outstripping progress. It has to be recognized that the potentialities of service are almost infinite and that escalating costs must limit what can be provided. Nevertheless, present services for children in this country fall short of what could and should be achieved. In this section, we consider some of the shortcomings.

Organization of services

In a country where there is a National Health Service it might be expected that guidance as to what the service is trying to achieve would come from governmental departments. In the UK this responsibility falls mainly on the Department of Health and Social Security and the Welsh Office in England and Wales, on the Scottish Home and Health Department in Scotland, and on the Northern Ireland Health Authority in Northern Ireland. However, from these departments there has been little or no leadership or movement towards integrating the child health service or towards developing and implementing national programmes in such fields as pre-school and school surveillance or the care of handicapped children, no drive to carry out the large-scale research needed in these areas, and no acceptance of organizational responsibility for appropriate training. These have all been left to the individual initiatives of professional organizations with resulting confusion of priorities in provision, patchy implementation, and the adoption of methods of unproven efficacy. At the regional and district levels there is frequently a lack of decision as to what, given the budget limitations, the priorities in child health should be; e.g. how much money should go towards hospital paediatric units, child health surveillance, and community support for handicapped children.

Responsibility for child health services at the district level varies from one district to another as between community unit managers, district medical officers, other specialists in community medicine, senior clinical medical officers, and consultant paediatricians with special interest in community child health. This unsatisfactory state of affairs is further complicated by the fact that the child health service crosses many other management boundaries, including those of the physiotherapy, occupational therapy, and speech therapy services, child guidance, family planning, community nursing, and so on. There has been failure of many Joint Care Planning Teams (see p. 160) to identify specific areas of child health need and, even when these are recognized, to make suitable financial provision for them.

Confidentiality of records
Parents often feel that they are not given enough information about the contents of their children's health records. Doctors vary in their opinions about the extent to which parents should have rights of access to these but nearly all would agree that the main determinant should be the child's best interest, a view expressed by the General Medical Council and the British Paediatric Association. The doctor's clinical judgement of what is best for his child patient is considered by the profession to be the proper basis for decision but there may be changes under the terms of the Data Protection Act (1986) which will define rights of access to computerized health records more clearly. While free interchange of information is the normal basis for consultation between paediatricians and parents, circumstances sometimes arise, particularly in respect of contraceptive advice to girls, where doctors and their child patients may be reticent about disclosure of facts and there may be a delicate balance between the parents' right to information concerning their child and the doctor's professional obligation to preserve confidentiality about the child's own disclosures. Parents already have greater access, following the Education Act of 1981, to information passed on to the educational services about their child's medical, psychological, and educational assessment. Parents should be able to see their child's immunization history (usually now available) and details of their child's pre-school and school health surveillance (which most parents at present do not see). While full parental access to health records information is unexceptionable in the great majority of cases, unrestricted access would worry a doctor who in the interests of the child wished for instance to record his suspicions on such matters as child abuse or neglect. In

such circumstances, however, it often proves more helpful to the child to discuss these suspicions openly with the parents at the time rather than to document them secretly.

These are matters of great complexity and some of the issues raised await further parliamentary clarification of the concept of limited access which seems to be the basis on which the Data Protection Act will be applied to computerized medical records. For the present, and probably for the future, the child's best interest will continue to be the most reliable guide in cases of doubt.

Prevention

Major obstacles to effective primary prevention are the continuing social inequality, poor housing, unemployment, and unequal access to health resources that prevail in this country at the present time. The number of children growing up in poverty is increasing as the gap between the rich and poor, in both income and health, widens (Smith 1986). However, while inequalities in health seem set to continue, it is essential that such preventive measures as are feasible are taken. Thus immunization uptake rates in many parts of the UK are not as high as they should and could be due, at least in part, to inadequate organization, ill-considered adverse media publicity, and lack of adequate campaigning effort. Health education in general could be more widely disseminated, though on the whole its methods are not well validated except by the occasional study; e.g. the finding that informing girls about the risks of rubella just before they take their consent forms home increases the uptake of immunization.

In many areas, genetic counselling services are not readily available. The basis of genetic prevention is accurate diagnosis followed by counselling by a clinical geneticist or physician experienced in this speciality. Advances in genetic diagnostic techniques in recent years have made it possible to prevent many defects and the number will increase in the future. The potential for prevention is great and genetic counselling with supportive services should be established under the NHS in every region of the country.

The hope that water throughout the country will one day contain adequate amounts of fluoride remains unrealized and dental caries is still far too prevalent amongst our children.

Research is required to validate screening programmes for the early identification of potentially handicapping conditions. A wider distribution of handicap teams and assessment centres is necessary because many secondary disorders in handicapped children remain unrecognized for too long and proper preventive measures are not instituted. All-important research is suffering through ever-tightening restrictions on university and NHS finances.

Health care

The changes which are gradually taking place in general medical practice give some grounds for optimism. Insufficient undergraduate education in child health and paediatrics and too little attention to community child health as opposed to specialist hospital care has meant that doctors were ill-prepared for family practice. This pattern is slowly changing and more appropriate undergraduate and postgraduate paediatric training should improve standards of paediatric practice in the future. Greater acceptance of team-work in primary care and the growing belief that family doctors, appropriately trained, should be responsible for maintaining the health and monitoring the development of children are trends justifying higher expectations. Militating against these developments are the dearth of adequate health care for some children in inner city and remote rural areas and the continuing reluctance of some doctors to perceive their role as other than responding to episodes of illness. Moreover, because primary health care services are organized on the basis of existing medical practices, which do not usually cover geographical areas, children are undoubtedly being 'missed'. The diminution in responsibility of health visitors for neighbourhood supervision has accentuated the risk of some children being overlooked, though this disadvantage has been more than offset by greater involvement of the health visitor in the primary health care team.

Nurses who are involved in child health surveillance, who provide follow-up nursing care for children whose specialized treatment originates in hospital, who help in the management of handicapped children, who undertake health education, or who work in schools require to be properly trained and experienced in children's nursing. Regrettably, this is by no means the case at present, as the importance of such training is not always fully appreciated and too often the expertise required for the nursing care of children is inadequately recognized or underrated.

With greater specialization and understanding of children's needs, the care of children in hospital in this country has improved substantially. However, despite increased awareness that admission to hospital is a frightening and disturbing experience for many children, and one to be avoided if possible, hospitals still admit too many children who could be treated on an out-patient or day-care basis. Many admissions are of course necessary yet, in spite of all the evidence and government direction that special hospital accommodation and facilities are necessary, many hospitals have no separate paediatric accommodation and children are still admitted into units not designed for them, or even into adult wards. This state of affairs has been tolerated for too long and is one of the most urgent matters facing the NHS.

Recognition of the emotional needs of children has fostered a growing trend to allow parents to stay with their children in hospital and also to involve them in an active participatory role in care. Further, there is a move to emulate the North American practice of building hotel-style accommodation close to large hospitals, so that parents and children can be together whilst lengthy investigations are carried out. These developments should be encouraged.

As in other spheres of medicine priorities have to be considered and funds allocated accordingly. Such forward planning as is undertaken too often evades essential decisions, which are made more difficult by new and unexpected demands. For instance, one of the more pressing problems facing the child health services is the increasing demand for specialized perinatal care. These services consume more and more resources in terms of money, staff, and equipment, yet the services provided fall far short of those required to provide adequate levels of care for new-born infants throughout the country.

Children with special needs

A group of children not well catered for by the NHS comprises those with special needs imposed by disability. Provision for such children has never been adequate, because from its inception the NHS was aimed primarily at patients with acute episodic disorders and those requiring 'crisis intervention' types of diagnosis, treatment, and management. The merging of the former local authority health departments with the NHS introduced a complementary element of community health care but the varied and changing requirements of children with continuing disability have not yet been adequately faced. There are a number of reasons for this. Formerly, children with serious disabilities were likely to die young, whereas now they can often look forward to a normal life span. Also the nature of continuing disability has changed over the years from mainly chronic illness, such as tuberculosis, rheumatic heart disease, and osteomyelitis, to predominantly neurodevelopmental disorders, such as mental subnormality, cerebral palsy, and spina bifida, which necessitate relatively less medical treatment but create demands for special education, physical therapy, promotion of social interaction, and preparation for a full and active life as an adult. The NHS was not designed to cater for such long-term needs, which are mainly of a non-medical nature but cannot be divorced from medical management and require some input of health service resources.

At a time when there is growing awareness of the deficiencies and attempts are being made to rectify them, new problems have been created by pressure to integrate handicapped children into ordinary schools rather than segregate them in special schools. This policy, laudable though it is, has led to the dispersal of scarce resources and expertise, especially in speech, and occupational therapy and in physiotherapy. Thus, whereas previously a therapist might see five or six children in a morning at a special school with all the required facilities close at hand, now much more time is needed to see the same number of children dispersed singly in various schools, often lacking necessary equipment. Although a recent survey showed that 65 per cent of health districts required increased resources to implement the integrative policy defined in the 1981 Education Act, no extra financial allocation has been made to education or health authorities for this purpose.

A further new factor is that many seriously handicapped children who would formerly have been in residential care for long periods are now looked after in the parental home and equipment costs have to be met in each case. An approximate estimate shows that a child aged one to two years, who is unable to walk because of cerebral palsy, will at that age require about £1000 worth of equipment. In a health district with 7500 births per year there may be 19 new cases of cerebral palsy, necessitating expenditure in the following year of up to £20 000, to say nothing of later needs.

Moreover, cerebral palsy represents only about 20 per cent of the total population of severely handicapped children.

Studies of handicapped children and their families have shown that there is a need for counselling, advice, and support to the families and, in later childhood and adolescence, to the children themselves. While much help of this sort is, or should be, given by members of the primary health team, social workers, teachers, and others, there is from handicapped families a widely expressed wish for someone less professional, more readily available and approachable, and with more time to devote to what often seem like trivial anxieties. Such counsellors may come from a variety of backgrounds but should have aptitude for the work and undergo training so that they give informed and practical advice and support in consultation with the professional advisers. There is a shortage of suitably skilled counsellors, which ought to be corrected as a matter of urgency. Some voluntary agencies are taking the initiative in this field.

These and other matters concerning the handicapped are considered in Chapter 4. The NHS does not satisfy the needs of the handicapped. The implications of providing for children with special needs are so great that only a new sense of priority and exigency and the allocation of additional resources can meet the needs and fill this large gap in the health services. Our society can hardly be considered 'civilized' if we do not make equitable provision for these children who, through no fault of their own, are so often condemned to endure unhappy and frustrated lives at a level far below their potential.

Voluntary services

The shortcomings in health services for children outlined above have stimulated much voluntary action to attempt to make good the deficiencies. Child care largely started in this way in the nineteenth century, with the activities of such people as Lord Shaftesbury and Dr Barnardo and of societies such as those founded by the churches, e.g. Waifs and Strays. The progressive development of statutory health services during the twentieth century, culminating in the establishment of the NHS, might well have been expected to render voluntary health work unnecessary. However, with the rapid advance of medical science and the limited resources of government, the need has continued and has led to the creation of numerous voluntary bodies in addition to the long-established agencies. Many of these new societies were started by parents of children with particular disorders and confine their activities to these. Their enterprise has contributed much but has resulted in some inequality in care and management in that some disorders with greatest need, especially mental handicap, do not attract as much support as their importance warrants.

A principal limitation of voluntary support is that it has no duty to meet every evident need. It thus tends to be unevenly distributed, often depending on the enthusiasm and industry of specific individuals. The statutory services, on the other hand, are required to provide for the whole population and the stretching of their limited resources to cover all who require them often means lower qualities of service. Further, in that different authorities often interpret their obligations in different ways, there are inequalities between regions and districts. The higher standard which voluntary societies may achieve may bring their statutory equivalent into disrepute. Such comparisons, while in some respects unfair, are useful in providing a yardstick for the statutory services: disparaging contrasts may be countered by establishing 'centres of excellence' within the NHS or local authority framework. Thus, while some voluntary adoption agencies (and also some local authority social service departments) offer services of a very high order, others fall far short of this optimum. To raise standards generally, sufficient new resources must be devoted to the work.

One way in which voluntary effort can provide for unmet needs is by developing the counselling and support services for handicapped children and their families referred to above. These are especially important at critical times in the life of a child with a disability: for example, when the implications of the handicap first become apparent to the family; when the child first goes to school; at adolescence—when the problems of independence, self-support, and relationships with the opposite sex assume such importance. Such counsellors must always work in the closest cooperation with the health professionals and others responsible for the care of the child, so that advice is based on sound information and does not conflict with anything the doctor or other adviser may have said.

Recommendations for the future

The basis of much childhood morbidity—social conditions, poverty, and their correlates—cannot be diminished by altering health services and therefore it may be thought that inequalities of health are so entrenched as to be irredeemable. However, much can be done to improve the health of British children by better health care and the best planning and deployment of resources. Here we examine some of the ways in which the child health services might be developed or changed to effect such improvement.

If money for the child health services were sufficient problems of apportionment would not arise, but it is not, so the question of priorities inevitably ensues. This implies detailed analysis of requirements and agreed planning decisions on relative merits and the allocation of funds. Even with such planning, however, an agreed programme may subsequently be disrupted by public pressure for some new form of therapy, regardless of how costly it is, how many will benefit from it, and how many others may be deprived by the consequent diversion of monies. Thus, for example, media publicity and demand for the provision of organ transplant facilities may pressurize a health authority into revising its priorities and postponing much needed developments in less fashionable services.

There are no wholly satisfactory answers to these dilemmas, for different individuals, professional and lay alike, will assess priorities in different ways and, even if consensus is reached, views may change in response to sudden new appeals. These difficulties are likely to intensify, as the complexity and cost of medical treatment increase and as, at the same time, the expectations of parents escalate. However, a major task and inescapable responsibility in the coming years will be to develop firm agreed plans which consider priorities and reconcile conflicting claims as far as possible and are followed by programmes of implementation which avoid unplanned diversions and remain flexible enough to respond to new valid demands. In this, central authority has an important role to play.

Planning of services

At the national level, there should be far clearer directives from the health departments on the rational organization of hospital in-patient and out-patient services for children, an agreed national screening programme as part of child health surveillance, and better central research planning into child health service requirements and priorities. Based on adequate national guidance and good information on the shortfall of provision within the areas of their jurisdiction, regional and district health authorities should formulate their own priorities for budgeting. This would enable those responsible for running the hospital, pre-school, and school health services and the services for the handicapped to determine priorities in their respective spheres. Lack of clearly defined objectives within regions and districts makes the planning of child health services extremely difficult.

Preventive services

Immunization uptake must be improved throughout the country by all available means, including better information for parents, nurses, and doctors on the indications and contra-indications of immunization, more convenient timing of immunization sessions, and greater use of mobile clinics. There is much to be said for the greater involvement of nurses and health visitors in immunization. Consideration should also be given to the question of making immunization mandatory for school entry.

With the greater relative prevalence of genetic and congenital disease in childhood, national, regional, and district clinical and laboratory genetic services should be better coordinated and expanded throughout the country, so that genetic counselling and facilities for prenatal diagnosis of genetic abnormality are readily available.

A more sustained effort to improve the environment of the most vulnerable families should be accompanied by vigilance to ensure that all children grow up in surroundings uncontaminated by noxious substances, including lead and potentially harmful radiation. Water should be fluoridated whenever the natural concentration falls below one part per million, so diminishing the need for dental conservation and releasing funds for other child health measures.

A national screening programme for neurodevelopmental disability and other disorders requires to be agreed between the professional bodies representing paediatricians, general practitioners, clinical medical officers, and health visitors. Such a programme, based on research data already available, should be instituted concurrently with a scheme for critical evaluation of the results. Each district must decide how best the programme can be carried out. The programme may well involve orthoptists, audiologists, and others as well as doctors, health visitors, and school nurses. Training standards should be specified nationally and appropriate training opportunities provided, particularly in the community child health service. All forms of evaluation will be greatly facilitated and simplified by the information now being collected under the terms of the Korner Committee's Fifth Report (Korner 1985).

Screening is of little value itself unless it leads to action, and adequate provision for subsequent assessment and ongoing management must be assured.

Health care

Neonatal care   Neonatal intensive care and special care units should have their own budgets so that the clinicians responsible can establish their own priorities and decide on the optimal use of their resources. In collaboration with the community child health services monitoring of the outcome for the infants treated in such units, in terms of morbidity as well as mortality, plays an important part in determining how many children will have special needs and the funds likely to be required to meet these. This, of course, will only partially indicate the size of the problem, since most childhood disability is not directly related to neonatal disorders.

Primary care   Appropriately trained general practitioners and health visitors should undertake health surveillance of children in their own practices, and all parts of the country should be covered by the primary care service. Appropriate training, both initial and continuing, should be organized and carried out utilizing academic departments of child health and consultant paediatricians together with senior clinical medical officers and suitably qualified general practitioners. Such training should figure more prominently in the training of medical undergraduates and trainee general practitioners. It is unfortunate that plans for improvements in undergraduate education, with greater emphasis on preventive medicine, family practice, and communication with patients, are being frustrated by the financial cuts which universities have suffered. The General Medical Council has recently warned the government that failure to maintain standards of medical education will adversely affect medical care into the next century.

Given sound training in child health and paediatrics, and continuing updating of knowledge, skills, and attitudes, the primary health care service should provide a comprehensive service for all children and the aim must be to raise standards throughout the country to those of the best practices.

Specialist paediatric care Specialization within paediatrics is likely to intensify in the future, both inside and outside hospital. Nevertheless, all paediatricians require some experience of general and neonatal paediatrics, community child health, and the care of handicapped children during their training. Every district general hospital should have five or more consultant paediatricians on its staff. At least three of these should work mainly in the hospital, undertaking general paediatrics usually with a special interest and expertise in some aspect, while at least two should be consultant paediatricians with special interest in community child health, working mainly outside the hospital. Paediatric consultants specializing in such fields as cardiology or neurology will be based at regional hospital centres and serve the needs of the whole region. Further thought should be given to concentrating highly specialized services in hospitals which serve a population large enough to maintain the skills and experience of the staff. This principle applies also to general hospital paediatric units, for small units do not treat sufficient numbers of children of different ages and with different disorders to afford their staff adequate continuing experience or to justify the trained paediatric nurses and the facilities and equipment needed for the care of infants and children. However well-intentioned the staff of a small unit may be, they cannot reach the standards of care that those in a large unit can achieve. High priority should therefore be given to ensuring that every child admitted to hospital goes into a unit intended for children and large enough to have staff and equipment attuned to children's needs. Parents who have to travel further to visit their children in hospital as a result of amalgamating small units into larger ones should have their expenses met as of right, thus offsetting one of the main disadvantages of concentrating in-patient resources.

Specialist child health services in the community should be more closely integrated with other children's services. Joint training programmes between health, educational, and social services at the district level would promote better understanding of the roles of different professionals. Therapy services for children, including physiotherapy and occupational and speech therapy, are often insufficient and are areas of potential growth; however, there has been little objective evaluation of the benefits derived from them and controlled trials should be instituted to assess the value of the techniques used.

There should also be careful evaluation of services for adolescents and of how best to cater for their needs.

Children in school

The school health service is an integral and important part of the child health services: every school should have a nominated school doctor and school nurse, who must have been appropriately trained. Specialist aspects of educational medicine are the concern of consultant paediatricians, particularly those with a special interest in community child health, and of specialist senior clinical medical officers. There should be sufficient numbers of doctors experienced in this field to ensure proper evaluation and care for every child with a learning disorder (BPA, 1987).

More emphasis should be placed on involving parents in discussion and communication between educational and health services about their children.

Teachers who have children with specific problems in their care should receive much better information and advice. This should be both by direct communication from the school doctor and/or nurse and through the availability of suitable written material.

Each school ought to have a defined policy about the administration of medicines and how these are kept in the school. This should include the role of teachers acting *in loco parentis* in such specific areas as giving drugs to children having epileptic attacks.

Health education should be included in the normal curriculum of every school and there should be more discussion and closer agreement on the best ways of achieving this.

Children with special needs

Large numbers, perhaps as many as 20 per cent, of infants and young children have or are suspected of having deviations from the normal course of development which may impose special educational or other needs in the future. The identification and assessment of such children is demanding of time and expertise. There should be agreed procedures of referral, which may vary from district to district. In general, each district should have a handicap team, led by a consultant paediatrician with responsibility for coordinating the assessment of children and for monitoring the sufficiency of therapeutic services and equipment for handicapped children in their district.

Not all children recognized by the primary health care team as requiring referral will necessarily need to be seen by the full district handicap team. In some areas children with lesser degrees of developmental deviation or only suspected of disability are referred to a small group, usually comprising a paediatrician and a nurse suitably trained for the work. Ancillaries such as therapists and social workers may also be involved. Such smaller groups should be established for every 100 000 of the population and may designate a member to visit the child at home. The needs of the child can then be discussed with the other members of the group, the family doctor and health visitor who referred the child, and the parents. If further referral is considered necessary the child may be passed to the district handicap team or alternatively by the family doctor to the consultant paediatrician in hospital, according to the particular need. In either case or, as often happens when the child is referred to the paediatric clinic in the first instance, the full resources of the hospital may be required for adequate investigation and treatment.

For children with serious disability, a wide range of provision should be available, since their needs vary so greatly. Each district should provide facilities for short-term respite care and make flexible arrangements for child-minding at home. There is a widespread need for better liaison and advance information about children with special needs who are either going to school for the first time or moving from one school to another. It is to be hoped that, in the near future, detailed research data will become available about the effects of the present policy of integrating children with special needs into ordinary schools, both on the children themselves and on the education and behaviour of the other children in their class and school. Matters requiring more research are (a) the effects on families, and especially on mothers, of the shift of handicapped children out of hospitals and other residential establishments and (b) the gaps in service provision as perceived by parents.

At all levels—district, regional, and national—the diagnostic and therapeutic requirements of handicapped children should be recorded together with the extent to which the necessary services and equipment are available and used. While the information must be considered in terms of the health service budget the aim must be that gaps in the provision of services are identified and filled.

At the national level, consideration should be given to devising a 'no-fault' compensation system, so that all families with handicapped children have the resources to achieve the best possible quality of life.

Conclusion

If the full potential of modern paediatric medicine is to be realized, more enlightened and more determined planning for integration and further development of the child health services is essential. Much could be achieved by redeployment and more effective use of existing resources. There must be better hospital provision for children, as well as more effective community measures for promoting child health. Inevitably this means greater expenditure of money, especially in areas like perinatal care. It is false economy to jeopardize the health of the next generation by according a low financial priority to such pressing needs.

Despite misgivings as to the extent to which these requirements will be met, there are grounds for cautious optimism about the future of the child health services. The NHS, with all its imperfections, does offer reasonably good health care to a large proportion of children in the UK. Doctors are increasingly working in group practice and in teams with members of other professions, including social workers, therapists and teachers, and, of course, health visitors and nurses. Efforts are being made to improve the exchange of information about children, with due regard for the confidentiality of records and the best interest of the child concerned. General practice and the community child health services are drawing closer together, and increasing numbers of family doctors, often working with clinical medical officers from the community service, are assuming responsibility for preventive as well as therapeutic primary care. The consultant and specialist services provide secondary care both in and out of hospital, including the specialized aspects of school health and educational medicine. More consultant paediatricians are bringing their expertise to bear on the problems of child health outside hospital, including long-term disease and continuing disability in children who attend hospital only occasionally.

These developments must be encouraged and facilitated. They are favoured by organizations well able to judge such as the British Paediatric Association, the Royal Colleges of Physicians, and the Royal College of General Practitioners. They are still viewed with suspicion by some community health staff. It is to be hoped that such differences of view, which have impeded progress towards integration of services, will soon be reconciled and that we can look forward with confidence to better health for our children in the years to come.

References

British Paediatric Association (1987) *Report on The School Health Services.*

Brotherston Report (1973). *Towards an integrated child health service.* Chairman J. H. F. Brotherston. HMSO, Edinburgh.

Court Report (1976). *Fit for the future: report of the Committee on Child Health Services.* Chairman: S. D. M. Court. HMSO, London.

Department of Health and Social Security (1980). Inequalities in health: report of a research working group. London DHSS.

Kilbrandon Report (1964). *Children and young persons, Scotland: report by the Committee appointed by the Secretary of State for Scotland.* Chairman: Lord Kilbrandon, Cmnd 2306. HMSO, Edinburgh:

Korner, E. (chairwoman) (1985), *Fifth report of the Steering Group for Health Services Information.* HMSO, London:

Sefi, S. and Macfarlane, J. A. (1985). Child health clinics: why mothers use them. *Health Visitor* **58**, pp. 129-30.

Smith, R. (1986). Whatever happened to the Black Report? *British Medical Journal* **293**, pp. 91-2.

7

Time past and time present for children and their doctors

ROY MEADOW

In the year before the sixtieth birthday of the British Paediatric Association (BPA) its sole surviving founder member, Bernard Schlesinger, died. Of today's paediatricians only a small minority had been born by the year in which their Association was founded, and they are in their last few years before retirement. The rest of us were born when the BPA was well established, even though many of us were in parts of the country where there was no formal paediatric service and no consultant paediatrician. None of us can look back critically at paediatric services during our childhood and compare them with those of today. We may have vivid memories of poliomyelitis, appendicitis, and diphtheria killing or maiming our friends, and we may remember the competitions at school to see who could spit gobbets of sputum the farthest, but recalling the detail of children's services is impossible; that time before the National Health Service (NHS) seems like a black-and-white newsreel, episodic and jumbled. The BPA came into being shortly after Joseph Stalin came to power in the USSR and Chiang-Kai-Shek in China. It was formed in the days of trams and the model T Ford car, long before the first use of sulphonamides or the discovery of penicillin. They were the days when the parish church was black, coated in honorable grime from the factory chimneys, and even from its tower no one could foresee that 30 years on the only tall chimney producing smoke would be the glinting steel stack of the new District General Hospital. The world and our society have changed more than the health services.

However, many paediatricians will remember vividly the children's wards and hospitals which they encountered as students and as junior doctors in the 1950's (Plate VI) and they can look back at what has happened to children's services during the second half of the BPA's life, that is, the last 30 years.

In 1958, and for some years after, there was still tremendous faith in the NHS. The British economy was growing, the NHS was expanding, and medical developments seemed limitless. My purpose is not to review the scientific aspects of medical progress during the last 30 years but rather to try and illustrate the way in which a changing society and a changing health service have made life for those working with children very different.

By 1958 most towns had a paediatrician who had duties at several hospitals and children's institutions. The cities and larger towns still had their children's hospitals, most of which had been built in the later years of the nineteenth century thanks to the generosity of wealthy local families. The London hospitals owed much to the Rothschild family (hence the proliferation of wards called after members of that family—Evelina, Lionel, and Charlotte) and to Siegfried Zunz, a metal merchant who endowed wards in memory of his wife Annie. Most were independent small hospitals which had an increasingly difficult time balancing their accounts until they were rescued by the NHS in 1947. Though many had a teaching hospital link few envisaged that they would be swallowed up by their neighbouring general hospitals and that so many wards, clinics, and staff devoted to children would be compressed into so little in the midst of large general hospitals whose main priority was not children.

The children's hospitals usually had a ubiquitous porter who was also the telephonist; he knew everyone in the hospital and the neighbourhood, the local families, the staff, and where to find them—who needed radiopaging and a bleep in those days? The other fixture was the lady almoner, a well spoken lady respectably dressed in twin set and pearls driving a Morris traveller. The similarity between her and today's medical social worker, in sandals driving a Citroën 2CV and overwhelmed by child abuse work, is difficult to detect.

Thirty or more years ago there were still a great many children's wards and many children in them (Plates I, II, and V). It wasn't just that rheumatic fever and other serious diseases were common but also that doctors and nurses relied on bed rest as a form of treatment. It was commonplace for a child with blood in the urine, believed to be the result of nephritis, to be kept in bed until the blood disappeared, and that might take up to a year. The average length of stay for a child with a medical condition was several weeks and, at the end of that time, as like as not, the child would be discharged to a convalescent home in the country or near the sea. Today the average length of stay is four days and convalescence takes place in the child's own home.

The wards were more likely to be designated for particular ages of children rather than for particular diseases, the only exception to that being separate wards for certain communicable diseases (in which cross-infection was taken much more seriously than it is today, all members of staff laboriously dressing up in gowns and masks and washing their hands for a timed period, using an egg-timer, before entering and leaving the child's cubicle).

The ward itself would have white tiles half-way up the high walls and at the top of the tiles a decorative tiled border. The floors were of polished wood and there would either be a big Victorian fireplace against the wall or a cast-iron stove in the middle of the ward (Plate I) with its chimney disappearing through the ceiling. There were not a lot of toys but there would always be a majestic rocking-horse and a large and beautifully kept doll's house some-times surrounded by potted ferns. The nurses knew the children well and they played games with them. There would be groups sitting round playing activity games, singing and clapping their hands, as one of the nurses looked after the wind-up gramophone. Some ward sisters lived in a room attached to the ward and were never really off duty at all for if there was a crisis they were called. The ward sisters knew the children best of all and some of them made it a rule to talk to every child for a few minutes each day on their own.

There were always a lot of pets about, and shoals of fish. In sister's office in a globe there would be very fat fish who received scones and sandwiches left over from tea, whilst in the main ward area there were ailing fish in large rectangular tanks containing a few bedraggled plants and a lot of rejected bricks, toy soldiers, and model cars. They were pale-yellow fish with mould growing on the abdomen and those that had been fed too many jelly babies and unwanted medications tended to float uneasily on the surface whilst the others laboriously flapped their tails hoping either to move across the tank or to shake off the long string of excrement that dangled down to the wreckage beneath. Elsewhere in the main ward area there were hamsters or mice revolving a wheel and, in a hutch out on the balcony, pet rabbits which all the children including those with asthma and eczema would cuddle and stroke. (An outbreak of fatal generalized vaccinia on a children's ward and the incrimination of the pet hamster, who had a chronic 'sore' on his tummy which the children stroked, was one of the reasons for the demise of pets from the ward.)

In some ways the children in hospital then looked healthier than today because children are only admitted to hospital today if it is essential and as soon as they begin to recover they go home. Whilst in hospital they are unwell and perhaps receiving unpleasant treatment or investigation. When that is complete they go home to continue treatment and recover. The staff do not have the satisfaction of well children running around, playing games, and being part of the ward community. Even in the 1960s it was rare to see an intravenous drip in a paediatric ward. When a child, for instance with severe burns, had to have a drip there was a special nurse beside the child monitoring the rate of flow. None could have imagined that portable infusion machines, with which the child could walk around, would be controlling intravenous fluids 20 years later. Nor could they have foreseen that the old Nightingale-style long open ward (Plate 1) would give way to a modern vinyl-floored, air-conditioned ward in a tower block, divided into small compartments and bays. Though a doll's house may be there somewhere it is overshadowed by posters of pop-singers and football stars, television sets, and computer games.

Feeding, meals, and potty training were taken seriously. What came out had to be as regular and regulated as what went in. On the toddler ward the children were sat in a great semi circle on their pots three times a day and left there until they performed. The smell lingers still in the memory and is a useful reminder that the modern District General Hospital has some advantages.

Ward-rounds

Doctors ward-rounds and particularly those by the consultant were a major event and engendered great respect from everyone. The children were in bed, in pyjamas, with the top sheet folded down the regulation 20 inches (Plate VI). Each child above the age of three years would have one colouring book and three crayons. Appropriate signs such as 'No Food or Drink' or 'Save All Urine' or 'Please Starve' (Plate VII) were attached to the bed. The consultant was not only able to find each child and receive an informed report on all from the senior nurse and the junior doctor but it was also quiet enough to examine the child thoroughly. When the consultant departed the atmosphere relaxed, nurses emerged from linen cupboards and went to work boiling up instruments in sterilizers to make up dressing trays which they set out on trollies, and the porter would trundle a stainless steel drum of sterilized swabs across the ward. The throw-away days of paper packs from the central sterile store were years away.

Consultants views were respected, perhaps too much; if one consultant was particularly upset by the sound of a child crying the canny ward sister would go on a reconnaisance before that consultant arrived and remove any crying baby temporarily into the linen cupboard. The ritual of the ward-round has declined for many reasons. An increased number of consultant paediatricians and a decreased number of child in-patients mean that no single consultant is responsible for as many children in hospital. The informality of the wards, the activities of play ladies, school teachers, and therapists, and the way in which children are playing around in their own clothes and no longer in bed (Plates IX, XI, and XII) has altered the practicality of a formal ward-round. Moreover, most ill children no longer have physical signs so that the story of the condition, the medical history, has become more important than the physical examination by the doctor, and that story is better followed and understood if everyone is sitting down in a quiet room or the doctor's office rather than standing in a group by a child's bed. Discussion of the child and family away from the bed has increased greatly and time spent on a ward-round by the bed has become relatively short. Moreover, if prolonged discussion with an older child or parent is needed it is likely that that will take place at the end of the round in an unhurried manner rather than in the middle of a ward-round with an embarrassed group of staff looking on.

Visitors

Perhaps the greatest change to the wards has been the advent of unrestricted visiting (Plates IX and X). As late as 1970 some children's wards had notices proclaiming 'Parents may visit on Saturdays and Sundays between 4 and 5 p.m.' Since many wards did not welcome telephone enquiries about children from their parents (and many parents were unfamiliar with telephones), the local evening paper gave information about the child's health in terms of 'critical' or 'satisfactory'—each child having a designated number so as to avoid publishing the name of the child. Parents gained access to children's wards slowly. Pioneers such as Sir James Spence in Newcastle and Dermod MacCarthy in Amersham created units in which mothers were encouraged to be with their ill children in hospital and look after them there. The National Association for the Welfare of Children in Hospital had an important political role in urging paediatricians and hospital authorities to allow parents more access, and in 1971 the government asked all hospitals to review their practices in relation to children and parents and asked how far the principles of the Platt Report (1959)—*The Welfare of Children in Hospital*—and the recommendations of the Department of Health and Social Security (DHSS 1971) had been implemented.

However, few could have foreseen the change that would occur within one child's childhood. Last winter the two children's medical wards at St James's in Leeds, which accommodate 56 children, had on one night 40 parents resident. [The current DHSS (1984) guidelines—*Hospital Accommodation for Children*—suggests that for every 20-bed children's ward there should be room for eight parents—the advice was out of date before the ink was dry.] Although modern wards have some mother and child cubicles the increasing number of resident parents means that most will be sleeping on mattresses on the floor beside the child's bed or on fold-up bed-chairs. Such a ward at night is a confused mass of bodies through which the night staff tread gingerly to reach the child. In the morning the ward kitchen is full of parents trying to brew tea or prepare their child's favourite cereal. Outside the treatment room mothers queue with trolleys to make up intravenous treatments which they will inject into plastic tubes and reservoirs attached to their child. The parents will be controlling the IMED infusion pumps and will already have attended to a fault by the time a nurse responds to the emergency failure alarm.

In the morning when the doctor comes round there is no neat bed containing a scrubbed, pyjama-clad child with colouring book and crayon—instead a dishevelled and tired parent asleep in the child's bed while the child, attached to a portable intravenous infusion machine, is in the playroom pressing the buttons of a computer game (Plate IX).

By the end of his round the doctor goes for lunch to the hospital canteen, a truly democratic place with no separate area for doctors or staff and accessible also to parents and visitors.

Life for the nurse on the children's ward is very different, and difficult. The nurse is no longer in complete control—she shares this with the parents. Parents always have known more about their children's feelings and behaviour than any member of the medical or nursing staff, but it is only recently that they have come to know more about their child's illness than some of the professional staff with whom they come in contact. For a child with a chronic or life-threatening disease the parents are likely to know more about the illness than the young nurse or, possibly, the recently qualified paediatric house officer, because they have had many discussions at the out-patient clinic with the consultants and they probably belong to a parents self-help group concerned with the particular disease and have read the informative literature provided by that organization. Those parents know a great deal about the disease itself and because they have had many brief recurrent visits to the ward they may also know the hospital and the ward rather better than the ever-changing junior staff. When the new nurse is looking for the linen cupboard or, in an emergency, for the resuscitation trolley such a parent is more likely to find it faster.

The insecurity of the young nurse working with experienced parents who are older than she is mirrored by the parents' comparable unease with the hierarchical staff in a large hospital. When the patient is very young the nurse is all too aware of the responsibility of caring for a frail and precious possession of someone else. With older child patients a young nurse may find it fearsome identifying closely with someone only a few years younger than herself who has a potentially fatal disease.

Ethnic minorities

For many paediatricians the largest change has come with the aggregation of different ethnic groups in certain cities. In some parts of these cities and in many towns more than one-third of the new-born babies are from a particular ethnic group; for instance, of parents originating from Pakistan. Because they tend to come from disadvantaged circumstances such children are frequent users of the paediatric services; the consequences are considerable.

Diseases are encountered that formerly were extremely rare (malaria has become more common than rheumatic fever or post-streptococcal nephritis). Dietary habits and different life-styles render them liable to different disorders but, above all, communication problems abound. A cynic would say that doctors and nurses, with their conservative backgrounds, have always failed to understand and to adapt in communicating with people from different or unconventional backgrounds. They certainly have great problems with those from different ethnic groups.

Although at home the Pakistani mother of a Muslim child may be more involved in mothering tasks than her white counterpart, when the child is ill she remains at home and the father brings the child to hospital and, in imperfect English, tries to give the history. Sometimes an elder brother or sister comes to act as interpreter. If the child is seriously ill the large extended family come along to support and sympathize, the women crouching on their haunches and, in periods of crisis, moaning beneath the dupatta or sari which they have pulled over their faces as a veil. It is a different picture to the traditional British stiff-upper-lip approach, and rather more understandable. The Muslim family may eat completely different food at home and require Halal preparation and cooking, but few hospitals oblige them. (It is interesting that some hospitals provide Kosher food for Jews, but not Halal food for the numerically more numerous Muslims.)

Neonates

In the early 1960s most new-born babies were looked after by the obstetricians and their staff; paediatricians were only allowed in by invitation. In 1961 as resident obstetrician at Guy's Hospital in London I was told by the consultant obstetrician to ask his permission before informing the paediatrician about a sick infant and, when that permission had been given, to write out a formal consultation request, put it in an envelope, and leave it in the front lodge of the hospital for the consultant paediatrician next time he came to the Hospital. But if the neonatal service was not geared for emergencies neither was our obstetric service, for my duties included caring for the hospital leeches—which thrived on placenta (the afterbirth)—and fulfilling the role of obstetric flying squad on a bicycle painted in the hospital colours with a midwifery bag on the handle-bars. By the mid 1960s a few neonatal units (for ill new-born babies) had sprung to eminence in Britain and, soon after, the rest of the country followed and neonates became a major part of paediatric work. Twenty years ago paediatric registrars seemed to spend much of their nights and weekends performing exchange transfusions and when they read of the work from Liverpool suggesting the likely benefit of anti-D rhesus immunization (see p. 258) they imagined that soon there would be little neonatal work left. Few foresaw the way in which neonatology, due to the large number of complex procedures which modern neonatal care entails (Plates XIV and XV), would become a major part of a paediatrician's work-load and one of the main reasons why consultant paediatricians get more out-of-hours calls to hospital than most other specialists. Some junior doctors are happiest in the neonatal unit, for there they can become skilled at difficult technical procedures and use them effectively to save lives and to benefit families, whereas, otherwise, at such a junior stage in their careers they could not possibly be as effective, or gain the same job satisfaction, dealing with problems of chronic illness or of psychosocial origin in the out-patient clinic.

Out-patients

New out-patient facilities have been in the forefront of hospital building programmes in the last 30 years. More patients attend out-patient clinics than are admitted to the hospital wards, and out-patient departments should have priority. The old out-patient departments or dispensaries for children were memorable and rather awful (Plates III and IV). Usually there was a large waiting hall with rows of bench seats. The walls would be decorated with Minton tiles depicting nursery rhymes, and off this main hall would be a succession of doors. From these doors rather officious looking nurses sallied forth from time to time. Within those doors there were usually a lot of people: the paediatrician, a senior nurse responsible for the patients attending that clinic, possibly a secretary, and a school attendance officer; and then trainees: a collection of medical students, physiotherapists, and nurses. It was virtually impossible for the parent or child to have a private conversation with the doctor. In some hospitals there were three or more doctors at different desks all in the same room each with their gaggle of attendants around them. One could hear not only what was going on at one's own desk but also at the others, and so could everyone else there.

The standard consultation was with mother and child. Sometimes grandmother came instead of mother, but it was rare for fathers to attend, and paediatricians of 30 years ago would have been amazed at the frequency with which today's fathers bring children to out-patient clinics and the great frequency with which both father and mother accompany a child to clinics. Then it usually was the natural mother or grandmother of the child who came to the clinic. Unemployment, shorter working hours, and, particularly, the larger role of fathers in the home and the child's care lead them to accompany the child to hospital and to join in the consultation with the doctor. But first of all the doctor has to ask the man with the child if he *is* the father because the complexity of family relationships as a result of the breakdown of marriage makes for much confusion. Today less than 5 per cent of children live in the standard story-book family of two dependent children, a father who goes out to work, and a mother who stays at home. The doctor no longer asks a mother about the health of her husband but rather about the health of his (the child's) father. It is usual to have to draw a family map to work out who lives at home, who the relatives are, who are the parents of each child, and the degree of relationship between the sisters and brothers of the patient—for so often they are half-brothers or stepsisters and often not blood relatives at all.

Today's out-patient suite is likely to be in a general hospital out-patient block. The facilities and rooms will be modern, there will be some toys around, but since the clinic is used for adult patients for more than half the time not too many structural alterations will have been made for the benefit of children and not too much equipment and play materials for children are left around. The parents will have more privacy because there will be far fewer nurses and staff in the clinic. It is unlikely the doctor will have a personal assistant or secretary in the consultation room. Medical or paramedical trainees attend clinics but they probably go there by rota so there will only be one or two students in the room, and then only for a small proportion of the clinics. It will be possible for troubled parents to be allocated a long time to discuss problems with the doctor and it is likely that the doctor will want to talk to them on their own without the child and also to the child on his own without the parents. The clinic no longer ends with the doctor dictating letters to his personal secretary; instead the ubiquitous dictating machine is there and he dictates his letters as he has a cup of coffee (for which his pay is debited £30.00 per year) at the end of the clinic. Sweets were common as rewards and bribes at the clinics of old but, in a hopeful attempt to disuade children from eating too much sugar, more hospitals will be using sticky labels and badges as a reward for coming to hospital or submitting to a painful procedure. It is probably a vain attempt because the waiting area outside the consultation room is occupied by a succession of overweight children all of whom are eating salted potato crisps and chocolate biscuits.

Festivals

Since many of the wards, and not just the children's wards, completed the day's activities with a hymn and prayers led by the ward sister it is not surprising that the hospital chapel of 30 years ago participated fully in all the religious festivals, with the child in-patients playing a prominent role particularly at the Harvest Festival and at Christmas.

Christmas itself had a strict ritual which all observed, many enjoyed, and in which some participated uneasily. On Christmas Eve the parish church choir sang carols in the ward. On Christmas Day the nurses wore their capes inside-out to display the red lining. In the hospital chapel at the main Christmas Day service, St John, Chapter 1, verses 1–14 was read by the medical superintendent and then the senior staff were dispensed sherry by matron in her hospital residence. A vast Christmas dinner was served on each ward. To this came all the staff who worked on the ward with their partners and children. The senior consultant carved the turkey in a grand manner and everyone looked as if posing for a Victorian Christmas card. The children who were still in hospital at Christmas (and there have never been a lot of children in hospital at Christmas because elective operations are not performed then and most families make great efforts to have their child home for Christmas) were somewhere in the background. The great Christmas tree and the lavish dinner were for the staff rather than the patients and as the presents were given out some of the staff felt a little uneasy that the presents were going to their own children rather than to the child patients—but then the patients had had their meal earlier and were tucked up out of the way in bed. The practice continued into the next decade but in more recent times these traditions have lapsed.

Radio and television commentators make occasional forays into children's wards at Christmas but find few patients there and staff who are unsure of what is happening. No longer are the senior doctors and nurses and the regular ward staff necessarily on duty on Christmas Day, and the seniors who rather uneasily come in with their families to wish those who are working a Happy Christmas find that those working are, because of shift systems and shorter hours, people whom they may not know. The Mayor, wearing his chain of office and leading his lady Mayoress, may still come round on Christmas Day but he has more difficulty than ever finding child patients to shake by the hand because the few who are in hospital are either too tiny or too ill to shake hands. Finding children to shake hands with the Mayor on Christmas Day has been a problem for a long time and even in the late 1960s paediatric registrars had to bring their own children into hospital to pose as patients to make the Mayor's visit worthwhile. [My daughter at the age of four years managed to shake hands with the Mayor five times in five different roles; as a surgical patient, an acute medical problem, a bed-ridden convalescent orthopaedic problem, and as a case of whooping cough (which she did extremely well for she had a horrible hacking cough).]

In the late-afternoon there was the hospital Christmas show, ostensibly for patients but really for the benefit of the staff. The jokes were in-service jokes with many references to notorious members of the hospital. The laughter and the singing came from the staff rather than from the few patients well enough to attend. On Christmas Day the hospital staff were congratulating each other on their good work and reinforcing belief in themselves and their institution. *Esprit de corps* and belief in an institution should not be sneered at; nor should they be adored, for institutions can create conditions that serve the workers better than the customers and the breakdown of those barriers may help patients to feel less fearful and displaced when they and their families have to be there.

The summer garden party and the autumn gift fair were similarly well supported by the hospital staff in times past. There was deference to rank and an expectation that the seniors would perform as if they were the local squires or nobility. There are still many fund-raising ventures for children's units, but how different they are! Groups of parents, many of whom have a child with a particular disorder, raise money to help children with that specific disorder. There are marathons and half-marathons with sponsored runners. Everything can be sponsored—at least one paediatrician found himself last year sponsoring nine children at one out-patient clinic to take part in a national record tap dance. There is everything from sponsored weight reduction to sponsored silence and those in the paediatric units sometimes feel a bit aggrieved at spending all their time at clinical or research work for children and then their money sponsoring their patients.

Expectations

Diagnostic labels with little meaning were common 30 years ago. They were even commoner 45 years ago when my mother who had a son with periodic bouts of tummy-ache and vomiting was well satisfied by the family doctor's diagnosis of 'acidosis' and the suggested remedy of regular drinks of orange juice with bicarbonate and glucose. But with increased diagnostic precision doctors, paradoxically, find themselves more often telling parents that they do not know the exact cause for a child's problem. On the one hand families demand truth and more information, but when they have it they are often disappointed. The imprecision of clinical diagnosis and the fact that therapeutic decisions have to be made on inadequate evidence are difficult for them to accept. The parents of a child who has had detailed investigation without a label being provided for the illness are likely to go off to a source of alternative medicine and to be impressed by the results of 'radionic box' analysis, a swinging pendulum, or alleged analysis of a piece of hair. They are given a precise label there and, perhaps more importantly, they get sympathy and a plan of action. The modern doctor's brutal honesty, in saying that there is no particular diet or tonic of proven benefit, does not suit parents who need to have something to do to help their child. Yet it has become more difficult to prescribe drugs in the 1980s. Though medicines and tablets are used less than they were 30 years ago the parents, because of media publicity, invariably ask about 'side-effects' and, as like as not, it

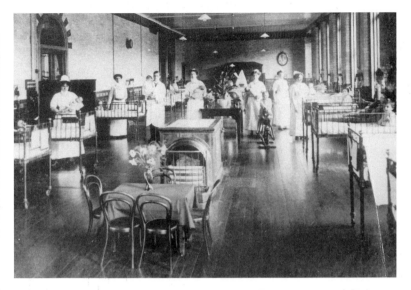

Plate 1 Pre 1914—a ward in a children's hospital (Hospital for Sick Children, Great Ormond Street, London).

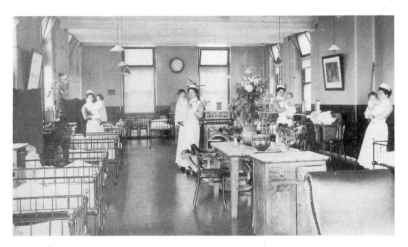

Plate II In the 1920s—a children's ward in a general hospital (St James Hospital, Leeds).

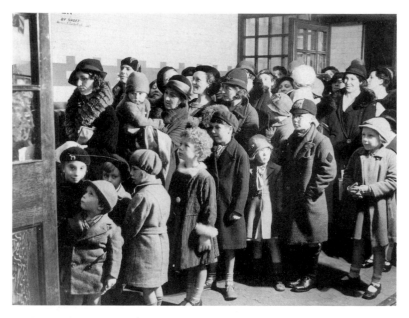

Plate III In the 1930s—queueing for admission to the Outpatient Department (Hospital for Sick Children, Great Ormond Street, London).

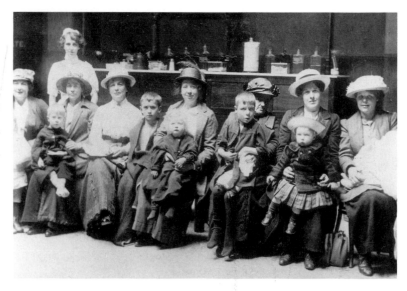

Plate IV In the 1930s—waiting in the Outpatient Department (Hospital for Sick Children, Great Ormond Street, London).

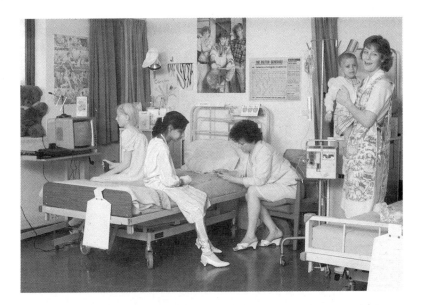

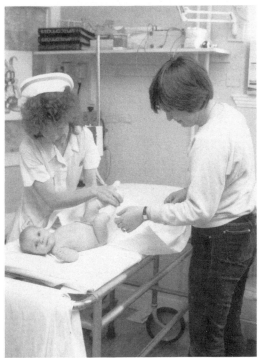

Plate IX (*above*) 1987—a corner of a children's ward in the same hospital as shown in Plate II. Unrestricted visiting for parents. The girl on the left, playing with a computer video game, has partial alopecia (loss of hair) from cytotoxic therapy and the coloured girl to her right is attached to that standard appendage of the 1980s: an intravenous line and infusion set.

Plate X (*left*) 1987— Mothers participate in the hospital management of their babies (Royal Hospital for Sick Children, Edinburgh).

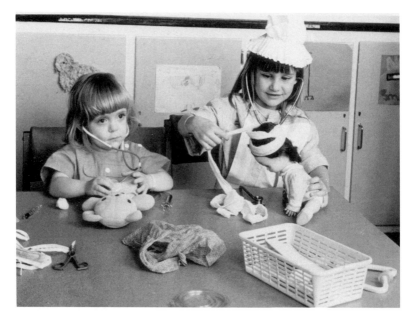

Plate XI 1987—The young ward doctors (Hospital for Sick Children, Great Ormond Street, London).

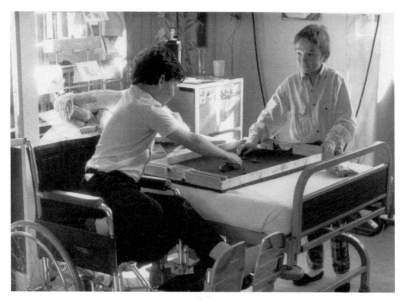

Plate XII 1987—'Your move' (Royal Hospital for Sick Children, Edinburgh).

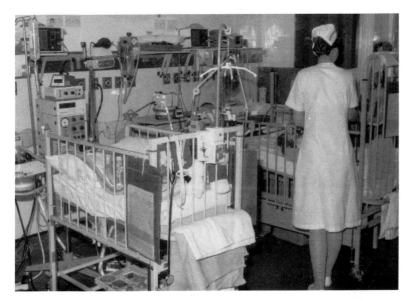

Plate XIII 1987—An intensive-care ward in a children's hospital (Royal Hospital for Sick Children, Edinburgh).

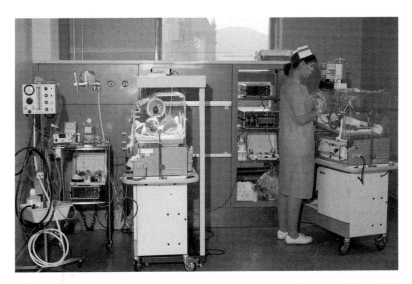

Plate XIV 1987—Ward in a neonatal intensive-care unit (Simpson Memorial Maternity Pavillion, Royal Infirmary, Edinburgh).

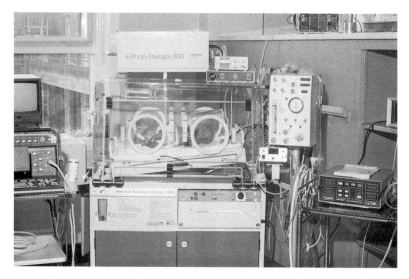

Plate XV 1987—Intensive neonatal care equipment. To the left of the incubator (containing a low-birth-weight infant) is a portable ultrasound machine, above the incubator is a phototherapy unit (for treating jaundice) and to the right of that an apnoea monitor (for detecting cessation of breathing): to the right of the incubator is a ventilator, above it, on the shelf, is a transcutaneous oxygen monitor (for measuring the oxygen content of the baby's blood through the skin without puncturing it), and below are an electrocardiograph and a blood pressure monitor (Simpson Memorial Maternity Pavilion, Royal Infirmary, Edinburgh).

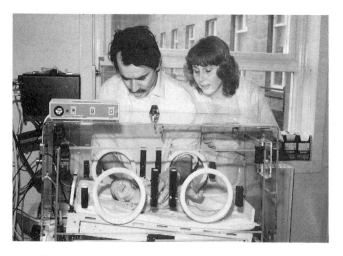

Plate XVI 1987—Parents handling their infant in a neonatal intensive-care unit (Simpson Memorial Maternity Pavilion, Royal Infirmary Edinburgh).

is the parent who has driven to hospital with the child standing on the front seat peering out of the sun-roof who then sits in the out-patient area stuffing his child with sweets before coming in to see the doctor and, with a flourish of his nicotine-stained hands, asks if the treatment that is being suggested has any 'side-effects'. The fear of side-effects from drugs contrasts with the facile acceptance of major surgery. 'Can't he have his heart operated on' says the mother of the child with a symptomless cardiac murmur. 'And if the blood doesn't go from the urine I suppose he could always have a kidney transplant' says the father, and the parents may even argue about which of them should donate the kidney, both wanting to.

Death is not accepted by doctors or parents any more. For doctors it is much easier to follow rigorous resuscitation policies and to carry on with technological procedures than to critically assess the option of death and the validity of withholding treatment. Those who have been selective about treatment in the past have rueful tales to tell of parents who agreed that the quality of life for their child with further treatment would be unacceptable and who therefore agreed that there should be no further treatment and that the child should die; but as the dying days came they then changed their minds and, as a father related, 'we acted like wild animals protecting our young' and sought treatment elsewhere. These problems will continue to cause profound diagreements and lasting unhappiness. One problem is that while adult patients can have the details of an illness explained to them, the odds for successful treatment calculated, and the consequences understood, and then give informed consent to a course of action, a child cannot. It is far from clear who should act on the child's behalf. In general it will be the parents, but as the Law Lords decreed in 1986 in relation to the Gillick verdict regarding the right of parents to confidential information communicated by their daughters to doctors the right to control a child on the basis of parental duty was

. . . a dwindling right which existed only insofar as it was required for the child's benefit and protection; that the extent and duration of that right could not be ascertained by reference to a fixed age but depended upon the degree of intelligence and understanding of that particular child and a judgement of what was best for the welfare of the child; that although in the majority of cases parents were the best judges of matters concerning the child's welfare, there might be exceptional cases in which a doctor was a better judge of the medical advice and treatment which would conduce to a child's welfare (Editorial 1986).

Most paediatricians feel profoundly uneasy about the exact situation which does justify the right to intervene against parental wishes; Yet at the same time they will be glad of the increased recognition of the individual child's rights as opposed to those of the parents. But inevitably when a child is desperately ill with negligible chance of worthwhile survival and the doctor mentions a new technique that might prolong life parents seize that chance; and if the doctor does not mention the new technique their neighbour probably will, for there will have been an over-optimistic account of it in the newspaper or the television.

Parents expectations of modern technical skill may be fulfilled but their need for more information and sympathy when their child is ill is rarely met. 'When your child is ill there is no such thing as enough information' said one mother 25 years ago (Meadow 1969), and perhaps that is the truth so that despite more time being spent explaining the nature and consequences of illness, the appointment of social workers and health visitors specializing in particular disorders, and the distribution of patient information leaflets, few families feel they have enough information when their child is ill— enough information is the ever-receding end of the rainbow. Unfortunately technical detail and explanation sometimes substitute for expressed sympathy and concern. Children and their families want someone to share their sadness with and someone to show that they care but few of the staff in a modern paediatric unit can satisfy those feelings.

Parents want explanation and unhurried time from the doctor, and they want it when they need it—urgently. However, their urgent need can compete with the urgent calls for the doctor to go to the Accident Department where a toddler has arrived fitting or to the new-born nursery where a baby has stopped breathing.

Technical aspects of medical care for ill children certainly have improved. Difficult procedures and difficult consultations are far more likely to be performed by a skilled and experienced doctor than they were. In 1962 as a locum senior house officer (SHO) I arrived in the operating theatre on the second day for the children's tonsils list and was told by the anaesthetist that the consultant did not come for that list and that the SHO operated. When I said I had never done the operation the anaesthetist said he would tell me what to do. That sort of occurrence would be impossible today. Skills are greater and a child in hospital will almost certainly be dealt with by staff who are experienced and competent with children. At the extreme end of high-technology medicine (Plate XIII) this results in a number of experienced senior staff devoting most of their time to a tiny number of children. A consultant paediatric nephrologist and several highly trained technicians and nurses may be spending three-quarters of their time with, say, 35 children. They look after them through the emergencies, the good days when the transplant seems to be working, and the bad days when rejection occurs and dialysis is needed again, and through the happier days when they will go off with a furniture removal van full of equipment for a summer seaside week to a holiday camp. That paediatric nephrologist is serving the children and families well, but what an extraordinarily high input of trained staff for so few children, particularly compared with the life of a consultant paediatrician 30 years ago, perhaps responsible for half a county.

The battered baby, prototype of all later forms of child abuse and neglect, had apparently not been born 30 years ago. But no-one today imagines that child abuse is a new feature of society: it has always been there and as society changes we are more willing to recognize it. However, those dealing with large numbers of abused children today do ponder about the surge of reported cases of physical, emotional, and sexual abuse. They still hope that this reflects society's unwillingness to tolerate child abuse but they cannot help wondering if there is not also a genuine increase of abuse, with children becoming even less valued in British society, and the stresses of unemployment and breakdown of family life leading to more abuse.

Envoy

Some things have not changed. Children continue to be prime clients for the general practitioner and take up 30–50 per cent of their consultations, yet the practice of children's medicine continues to occupy only 5 per cent of the medical students' timetable. Though children comprise 20–25 per cent of the population they still lack a strong political voice nationally, and in medical politics there are few who speak up for them. Most of the powerful barons of medical politics understandably put the needs of their main clients, adults, first. The steady loss of children's hospitals has made this more serious. It is not the loss of Minton tiles, fish-tanks, lady almoners, Peter the porter, scones in sister's office, or institutional festivals that should be lamented, for as they disappeared children's units became less institutionalized, more accessible to families, and much more effective in their medical care. The real loss is of the power that a children's hospital had for children's services. For in a children's hospital there was never doubt that children came first, but once those wards had been compressed into large general hospitals the children lost their voice and their pre-eminence forever.

References

DHSS (1971). *Hospital facilities for children* HM(71)22, Department of Health and Social Security. HMSO, London.

DHSS (1984). *Hospital accommodation for children.* Health Building Note 23, Department of Health and Social Security. HMSO, London.

Editorial (1986). *Arch. Dis. Child* **61**, pp. 725-6.

Meadow, S. R. (1969). The captive mother. *Arch. Dis. Child* **44**, pp. 362-7.

Platt Report (1959). *The welfare of children in hospital.* Chairman: H. Platt, Department of Health and Social Security. HMSO, London.

8

Ethical issues in child health and disease

A. G. M. CAMPBELL

Only one rule in medical ethics needs concern you—that action on your part which best conserves the interests of your patient (Martin H. Fischer 1879-1962).

Introduction

Until relatively recently few paediatricians, or any other doctors for that matter, gave much thought to the moral judgments implicit in clinical decisions. Their practice was influenced by their personality, training, cultural and perhaps religious upbringing, and by their understanding of various codes of professional ethics to which they might have heard vague reference at medical school. Paternalistically, they took for granted that their decisions and actions were always for the good of their patient, and the 'rightness' or 'wrongness' of a decision in moral terms was rarely questioned either by them or by others. Indeed it is doubtful if 'medical ethics' to most doctors meant more than advertising, poaching patients, improper relationships with patients, or various matters of professional etiquette. They probably gave even less thought to ways in which their work in caring for sick people might bring them into conflict with the law.

All that has changed. During the past two decades 'biomedical ethics' has become a fast developing growth 'industry', although codes of ethics to guide doctors in the practice of medicine have existed for over 2000 years (Etziony 1973). The bibliography is rapidly expanding; ethics research institutes have been established in several countries including the UK; most professional organizations have ethics committees; and 'hospital ethicists' have been appointed in the USA. For individual paediatricians it may seem at times as if almost every major clinical decision is subjected to ethical analysis or legal scrutiny, perhaps by individuals not even remotely connected with the child or family.

One major impetus to this ethics explosion was the catalogue of Nazi atrocities exposed at the end of the Second World War. Particularly appalling for the medical profession were revelations about the doctors who violated the basic tenets of medical ethics by conducting medical experiments that infringed human rights and all sense of human decency. The Nuremberg Code subsequently established basic principles to govern the conduct of human research '...in order to satisfy moral, ethical and legal concepts'. The first principle states that 'The voluntary consent of the human subject is absolutely essential', a requirement that is impossible to achieve in infants and young children and one that continues to trouble paediatricians today[1].

A second reason for the growing visibility of ethical issues in medicine is the remarkable change that is taking place in medical practice itself. This is seen to most dramatic effect in our ability to control life and death. Embryonic life can be created in the laboratory; the life of an individual can be prolonged, sometimes it seems almost indefinitely; and the timing and manner of death can be changed. This awesome assumption of power over life and death inevitably has created new ethical dilemmas for which traditional codes are seen as increasingly inadequate. Even new definitions of death have been necessary and newer ethical codes and principles have been enunciated in attempts to keep up with these developments. Like the Nuremberg Code others have addressed the problems of research, notably the World Medical Association's Declarations of Geneva in 1948 and of Helsinki in 1964 (revised in 1975 and 1983). Some codes are issued by national organizations and addressed to specific professional groups, some address specific topics of current concern such as 'brain death' or 'the care of handicapped infants', and as if to illustrate the changes in doctor/patient relationships the American Hospital Association has issued a patients' Bill of Rights. This reflects the replacement of paternalism in medical decision-making by a more contractual form of agreement in which patient autonomy is given primacy.

Recent codes or guidelines are attempts to reflect, not always successfully, a rapidly changing practice of medicine in a rapidly

---

[1] See Appendix I and II for extracts from modern ethical codes or guidelines.

changing society—new knowledge, new skills, new technology, new working relationships, new organizational structures all taking place against a background of increasing public attention and demand for accountability, not just to patients and families but to others including the State. Increasingly a doctor's duties and responsibilities to society may come into conflict with his primary obligation to act in the best interests of his patients and to safeguard their dignity as human beings. It is tempting for an individual doctor to avoid complex ethical issues and to concentrate on the easier technical problems of delivering care, a temptation sometimes difficult to resist when so many doctors now function as members of a multidisciplinary team. While this may be the easy way out for a doctor it may constitute an abandonment of patients at times of greatest need.

For paediatricians the dilemmas are particularly difficult and poignant as child patients cannot exercise autonomy and participate in decisions that vitally affect their future. We generally accept that parents will make the major decisions affecting their child and almost always will make them in the best interests of the child and the family. Paediatricians also regard themselves as advocates for children usually in partnership with parents but occasionally in conflict.

Ethics and the British Paediatric Association (BPA)

Like other organizations the BPA first became involved in ethical issues through concern about the involvement of children in research. How quickly ethical thinking has changed in the past 20 years can be gauged from this extract from a minute of the BPA's Academic Board Meeting on 7 December 1968:

93 (89) *Ethics of research investigations in children*
  The chairman (Professor D V Hubble) presented a paper written after discussions held by the Working Party. It was agreed that the paper was a valuable contribution which set out most of the problems and arguments. However it was obvious that members could not reach complete agreement on a subject which involved individual ethical practice and it was decided to file the paper and take no further action.

The matter was debated again in October 1972 in response to sporadic letters from paediatricians expressing concern about the lack of authoritative guidelines for research:

'It was decided that the original decisions of the Board still held good. These were that the matter of ethics and research in children was too complicated and too much a matter for personal decision on the part of the doctor to lay down even the simplest of guidelines. It was felt that attempting to do so might even inhibit the progress of research on children and that perhaps the best guides to proper practice were the attitudes of mind of the researcher and the approval of his colleagues' (Academic Board Minute, 14.10.72).

Although the question continued to crop up from time to time it was not until January 1978 that the Academic Board requested the BPA's ruling body, the Council, to set up a Working Party 'to draw up a brief document stating the case for research on children and giving examples of instances where major benefits for child care had resulted from such research'. (Executive Committee Minute, 20.1.78). The Working Party consisted of Dr A. D. M. Jackson (Convener), Professor F. Cockburn, Professor J. A. Dudgeon, and Dr D. M. T. Gairdner. Their report was approved by the BPA Council in May 1979 and published the following year (British Paediatric Association 1980).

At the same meeting the BPA Council agreed that a Standing Ethical Advisory Committee be established 'to meet on an *ad hoc* basis in response to requests for advice from local ethics committees'. Apart from its first convener (Professor F. Cockburn), the Committee consisted of the Chairman of the Academic Board, a nominee of Council, and a representative of the British Association of Paediatric Surgeons (BAPS). Thus the current BPA/BAPS Ethics Advisory Committee grew out of the need to clarify the ethics of research—'the function of this Committee will be to offer advice on the ethics of research projects involving children'—but its advice is now sought on a wide range of ethical issues of importance to children and paediatricians. With most of these troubling dilemmas where each individual will take different moral positions it is difficult to reach complete agreement and often impossible to state any 'official' BPA view that will achieve universal acceptance. Nevertheless the BPA recognizes that if it is to maintain leadership in its advocacy for children it must be prepared to give some guidance to members (and the public) on the issues that increasingly concern them.

Life, death, intensive care, and the problem of severely disabled infants

In 1981 paediatricians became uncomfortably aware of the glare of publicity and public debate about the care of handicapped infants when the late Dr Leonard Arthur, at the instigation of 'Life' (a self appointed organization which purports to protect life) was accused and subsequently tried and acquitted of murder at Leicester Crown Court. Paediatricians were uncomfortable because they recognized that some of the accusations levelled at Dr Arthur might just as easily have applied to them and that Dr Arthur's decisions in the management of John Pearson raised difficult moral and ethical questions about the acceptable limits of paediatric practice. The debate was not new but had received increased attention with the development of new treatments and modern intensive care. Franklin discussed the issues sensitively in 1963 when he dealt specifically with the problems raised by infants severely handicapped by thalidomide and indicated that 'We have to work towards the baby's acceptance by the family and by society. This means maximum possible aid for the baby'. Later, however, he admitted that 'if the baby has a lethal lesion I am not sure that we are always inevitably bound to full treatment. In this case the parents should never be drawn into the discussion' (Franklin 1963). Illingworth and Illingworth (1965) also stressed that 'with the rarest of exceptions, the severely defective child should be treated in exactly the same way as the normal child' and prophesied that if not 'there will be constantly recurring ethical problems and doubts; and more important than everything else, mistakes in judgment will sooner or later be inevitable'. Others took a very different view: 'The save-all policy has become the rule in our obstetric and paediatric services, with results which could become grave in terms of human suffering' (Slater 1971). Lorber (1971), reviewing the results of the Sheffield policy of routine operative closure of all meningomyeloceles (severe spina bifida), implied that it would be wiser to be more selective and leave the more seriously affected children unrepaired in the hope that they would die and be spared lives of considerable suffering and handicap. A similar debate was developing in the USA, and in 1973 considerable publicity was given to two articles which for the first time documented the significance of these difficult dilemmas in the context of modern neonatal intensive care (Duff and Campbell 1973; Shaw 1973).

Doctors have a clear commitment to respect life. Nowhere has this been more evident than at birth and in the early weeks of postnatal life. Almost 100 years ago, Pierre Budin, the French obstetrician, who deserves most credit for first demonstrating the benefits of 'new-born special care', showed that by keeping premature babies warm he could achieve a remarkable improvement in survival. But even Budin recognized that there were limits: 'We shall not discuss infants of less than 1000 g, they are seldom saved and only very rarely shall I need to allude to them' (Budin 1907). Until the 1950s and the development of modern intensive care the high mortality continued among premature and abnormal infants. It was accepted with an 'its probably just as well' attitude that reflected not just medical or surgical impotence but professional and parental concern about these infants' prospects for future health and the likely impact on the family. There was little attempt to keep them alive, and in the privacy of the home, and even in the hospital delivery room, death may have been hastened to avoid more prolonged suffering. Parents grieved for their loss but most were able to celebrate the birth of a healthy infant in subsequent years. It is worth noting that the still-birth rate for spina bifida fell considerably after the introduction of a more optimistic approach (Forrest 1967).

Fortunately most infants treated in a modern intensive care nursery (Plates XIII, XIV, and XV) grow up to be healthy or to suffer from only minor disability. A few survive with grave handicaps that have serious consequences for them and their families. Three groups of infants are usually affected: very-low-birth-weight (VLBW) infants who are surviving premature birth in increasing numbers at earlier and earlier stages of gestation; infants who have been severely brain damaged by some complication of pregnancy or birth such as infection or asphyxia; and infants with major and multiple abnormalities, particularly those involving the brain.

Arguments about the appropriate care for these infants are focused on three broad options. *First*, the moral obligation to respect and preserve life as enshrined in the Hippocratic Oath commits doctors to treat all infants equally whatever their condition and future quality of life. Efforts should be continued to provide all necessary treatments to maintain life, including the surgical correction, where feasible, of life-threatening abnormalities. This is the view expressed by various 'right to life' organizations and is reflected in the 'Baby Doe Rules' recently introduced in the USA.

Second, where there is a high likelihood of severe disabling handicap, particularly involving the brain, medical treatments apart from those necessary to relieve distress may be withdrawn or withheld after discussion with the parents and usually with their agreement. In other words, these infants should be allowed to die. This option, or variations of it, is favoured by many paediatricians, is supported by most parents who face these tragic dilemmas, and, as far as can be judged, is accepted by the general public.

Third, some philosophers, but probably very few paediatricians, consider that, while death may be preferable to life clouded by handicap, to allow an infant to die is morally no different from killing. They argue, however, that to take positive action to end life quickly and painlessly, although currently illegal, would be more humane and morally more defensible than allowing a child to die perhaps slowly and painfully.

Doctors confronting these dilemmas soon become aware of how traditional codes have failed to keep pace with changes in medical practice and contemporary society. As one philosopher stated, 'The old answers will not do any more; they were made for other times and for other places' (Ladd 1980). In attempting to set guidelines, as the BPA felt necessary in 1982, it soon became obvious that paediatricians, like others, all view the issues in different ways. Only very general guidelines were possible with considerable latitude being left to individual doctors caring for individual infants in individual families with individual circumstances. Where questions of morality are concerned we all tend 'to draw lines' at what we believe to be right or wrong and hope they conform to the ethical standards of our profession and of the society in which we live. We must also be aware, and may need to make parents aware, of where our actions may stand in relation to the law. The fact that we might view an action as moral does not necessarily make it legal, and an action we as individuals might view as immoral could nevertheless be perfectly legal.

Infants of very low birth-weight
Like Budin, we used to consider 28 weeks gestation age (term is 37–42 weeks) as the limit of viability for an infant born prematurely.

Nowadays infants born between 24–28 weeks have a good chance of survival and occasional 'successes' have been reported under 24 weeks. Unfortunately while the prospects for the larger and more mature babies are reasonably good, for infants under 26 weeks (or under 800 g) the risks of severe disabling complications with future handicap increase significantly. Should all infants born alive be rescued to the best of our abilities and without regard to the consequences for the child and family or should a line be drawn somewhere? It is only relatively recently that some have begun to look on the salvage of *all* viable babies as a desirable social goal:

> The history of efforts to accomplish this ideal has been marked by continuous conflict because the attitudes of parents have not always been congruent with the views of authorities. A recurring question has been, 'Whose baby is it anyway?' (Silverman 1981).

Elsewhere I have suggested a 'cut-off' birth weight of 750 g below which the likely outcome and future implications with or without treatment should be discussed with the parents before various resuscitative and intensive care procedures to maintain life are continued or introduced (Campbell 1982). It must be emphasized that a 'cut-off' weight only makes sense if it is flexible and considered as only one of a number of criteria that should be considered carefully before coming to any decision. Maturity (gestation age), the condition of the infant at birth, especially the vigour of spontaneous breathing efforts, and absence of other complications or abnormalities will obviously be important. Many neonatal units use these or similar criteria, but some, because of different or conflicting moral views, or perhaps because of anxiety about the legal implications, continue to treat all infants aggressively from birth, even those weighing as little as 500 g or less. In practice, most doctors will initiate aggressive treatment, including intubation and assisted ventilation, for all infants who seem potentially viable, to give them a 'trial of life', but if further events or later assessments indicate that there is a high likelihood of brain damage, treatment will be stopped and the infant allowed to die. What part parents play in reaching these various decisions is difficult to assess but from published accounts paediatricians seem increasingly willing to discuss the options for care fully and frankly with them and to seek their views before making any final decision. New medical skills and technology along with careful follow-up studies of the survivors will dictate continuing changes in criteria. They will also vary from country to country and from nursery to nursery according to the resources available. Unfortunately increasing pressure to modify criteria according to resources will become a fact of life. Instead of ignoring these constraints paediatricians should ensure that setting such criteria will remain their responsibility.

The severely damaged or malformed infant

Parents are concerned about what an abnormality, especially 'brain damage', means for their child's future health, happiness, school, normal relationships, and future independence—what Rachels (1986) calls 'having a life' as opposed to merely 'being alive'. This is a most important distinction and is undoubtedly a major factor influencing paediatricians in advising parents. Specific examples include severe perinatal asphyxia, congenital virus infection, and severe forms of spina bifida with hydrocephalus. There are also a number of chromosomal disorders with multiple abnormalities that are almost invariably associated with mental handicap. In some of these, e.g. trisomy 13, the infants are so grossly deformed that anything like an acceptable life is impossible and early death is likely in any case. On the other hand, Down's syndrome (trisomy 21), the best known of the chromosomal disorders, is in a very different category and has been the subject of many ethical and legal controversies.

Allowing to die—taking the decision

Most doctors reject absolute adherence to the sanctity of life as inhumane vitalism that takes no account of tragic errors in development, the realities of disease, or human suffering. At the other extreme they are wary of suggestions that the swift painless killing of severely deformed or brain-damaged infants would be more humane and should be sanctioned by law. Paediatricians generally prefer an intermediate position which recognizes that in certain circumstances withholding or withdrawing life-preserving treatments and allowing the infant to die would be best for the child, for the family, and probably best for society. There may be no *moral* distinction between 'killing' and 'allowing to die' but there is a powerful *psychological* distinction which is important to the staff of intensive care units. To them there *is* a big difference between not using a respirator to keep an infant of 600 g alive and giving a lethal injection, although the end result is the same. There may be hypocrisy in this but there are times when a certain amount of hypocrisy is necessary.

Within this intermediate position or 'grey area' there will be considerable differences in individual moral reasoning to make a treatment or a no-treatment decision acceptable or unacceptable. It must be remembered that the parents who (apart from the child) are most affected may also take very different positions. Doctors must be careful not to impose unwelcome choices on families or create conflicts within the families through a sense of moral superiority, yet they may have to guide them towards what is acceptable, not only medically but morally and socially, and what is within the law. Thus much latitude in decision-making must be expected and should be tolerated. Occasionally the parents' understanding of the medical realities and their views on the options available may be so faulty that disagreement will result and it will be necessary to seek court assistance in order to proceed with urgent treatment. Parents may occasionally ask the doctor to 'do something' to hasten death in the severely handicapped infant whose prolonged dying is causing great anguish. While such an action might be viewed as morally correct, the parents must understand that it would be against the law and that there might be legal consequences for them as well as for the doctors.

Baby Doe, government involvement, and infant-care review committees
The intolerance of 'right to life' activists in the USA has forced the US Department of Health and Human Services (DHHS) to restrict latitude in decision-making. In May 1982 the DHHS informed hospitals in receipt of federal funds that under Section 504 of the Rehabilitation Act of 1973 it is unlawful

... to withhold from a handicapped infant nutritional sustenance or medical or surgical treatment required to correct a life-threatening condition if (1) the withholding is based upon the fact that the infant is handicapped; and (2) the handicap does not render treatment or nutritional sustenance medically contra-indicated.

This warning was the forerunner to attempts at legislation which came to be known as the Baby Doe Rules after a controversial and well-publicized decision in Indiana to withhold life-saving surgery from an infant with Down's syndrome, known to the public as Infant John Doe. This legislation was intended to prevent paediatricians, in consultation with parents, from exercising discretion in the use of intensive care and other life-prolonging treatment. Paediatricians, who devote their professional lives as advocates for children, now found themselves under suspicion as potential if not actual murderers. These 'ill-considered proposals' were attacked by many individuals and medical organizations, including the American Academy of Pediatrics (AAP) but the DHHS persisted in its determination to outlaw 'quality of life' criteria for the care of handicapped infants in spite of a series of legal defeats culminating in the final rule being declared 'invalid, unlawful and without statutory authority'. It was pointed out that Section 504 of the Rehabilitation Act applied only to issues of education, employment, and transportation and not to medical decision making.

Following these legal defeats the DHHS adopted a new tactic. It brought 'withholding of medically indicated treatment' within the legislation on child abuse and called it 'medical neglect', a move that families and paediatricians, acting sincerely in infants best interests, found particularly offensive. The amendment to the Child Abuse Prevention and Treatment Act came into effect in October 1984. This requires individual States to set up their own procedures for dealing with reports, that can be made anonymously by anyone, of failure to provide treatment. The amendment defines this as

... all treatments likely to be effective in ameliorating life-threatening conditions except:
1. When the infant is 'chronically and irreversibly comatose'.
2. When the provision of treatment would:
   (a) Merely prolong dying.
   (b) Not be effective in ameliorating or correcting all of the infant's life-threatening conditions, or
   (c) Otherwise be futile in terms of the survival of the infant.
3. When the provision of such treatment would be virtually futile in terms of the survival of the infant and the treatment itself under such circumstances would be inhumane.

Fortunately these definitions give much more flexibility and discretion, but it is perhaps inevitable that American paediatricians continue to feel extremely vulnerable to legal intervention and possible penalty, and not surprising that more infants are now subjected to excessive, cruel, and pointless prolongation of suffering.

Parents, who have to bear the consequences of these decisions influenced by government dictate, were almost completely ignored by the drafters of the Baby Doe Rules (Angell 1983). One can readily understand if their sense of injustice was particularly acute in a society whose government, at the same time as introducing this legislation, was also threatening to reduce the funds available for the care of handicapped persons in the community.

The most significant result of the American Academy of Pediatrics opposition to the legislation was agreement that hospitals might set up their own Infant-Care Review Committees (ICRC) with professional and lay membership to guide hospital policy and advise on individual problems, thus acting as a buffer between the doctors and State intervention. These committees are now operating in most major hospitals but their impact on medical decision-making remains unclear. Certainly, in some respects, they seem to be successful but it is more difficult to know if they have led to 'better decisions' for individual families (Fleischman 1986).

In the United Kingdom there is no legislation similar to Baby Doe although there were calls for it after the Arthur case. On the contrary, a Limitation of Treatment Bill was proposed which, with appropriate safeguards, would allow the killing of severely abnormal infants up to 28 days after birth (Brahams and Brahams 1983). While this Bill would provide some legal protection to paediatricians and might remove some of the absurdities of the present distinction between the legal killing of fetuses and the illegal 'killing' of new-born infants, many are reluctant to see State involvement either to enforce life or to dictate death. Some modification in the current law is desirable but there is some merit in doctors and parents continuing to trust each other in agonizing over the dilemmas and debating the issues with care. Legalizing a form of infanticide might erode much of this trust. What parents and doctors need from those in society who would harshly condemn quality of life decisions in moral terms are more understanding of the injustices of biology, more compassion for the afflicted infants, more appreciation of family realities in individual circumstances, and considerable latitude to work out the dilemmas in the best interests of the infant and family. Deciding to withhold or withdraw treatment to allow a child to die may be viewed as immoral by some and illegal, even murder, by others, but for the child and family it may be the least detrimental of a number of unsatisfactory options. For us all it is a dilemma that must be faced no matter how troublesome. Deciding to keep all infants alive using any skills and resources available without regard to the consequences while all the time pretending that there is no decision to make is a devastating decision of default. It may be the easier way to avoid difficult moral questions but it diminishes the role of the doctor to that of a technologist, skilled in techniques but devoid of compassion. Instead of remaining its masters we become the servants of a rapidly expanding technology running out of control.

'Family-centred' neonatal care

In my view the main burden of these decisions must continue to be borne by the doctor or doctors primarily responsible for the infant's care in conjunction with the family, primarily the parents. Doctors and parents will both seek advice from others. The doctor will consult with colleagues to ensure accuracy of diagnosis and prognosis; with nurses who provide the consistent hour-to-hour care and often come to know the parents intimately at the cot-side; and with others who function as part of the intensive care team. The parents may seek the views of grandparents, clergymen, friends, and perhaps many others. As reflected in national and cultural differences, some parents will still prefer to leave much or all of the decision-making to doctors, trusting them to act in their baby's best interests as they have done for generations. This pattern of decision-making has been described as 'family-centred' because families are most familiar with their own strengths, weaknesses, and resources and must bear the consequences of any decision (Duff and Campbell 1976). Lawyers have criticized the lack of 'due process' in such a policy and have pointed out the legal dangers to paediatricians (Robertson and Fost 1976). Up to a point, lack of legal due process is a valid criticism but the problems of individual infants interacting with family circumstances may lead to complex and almost unique situations for which only general guidelines can be provided. The medical prognosis should not necessarily be the only determinant. There must be some room for discussion based on values cherished by individual families—personal, religious, and cultural. We have been resistent to outside interference in these tragic and intensely private affairs unless there are clear abuses of trust or if harm is being done to someone. It is important that the decisions are made openly and that doctors are held accountable. They must be prepared to defend their decisions in court if necessary. Committees can provide valuable objective analyses of the issues and can suggest policy guidelines but like armchair ethicists, philosophers, and lawyers they can only be peripheral to the individual tragedies.

Rhoden (1986) calls the family-centred approach an 'individual prognostic strategy' and believes that it is

. . . most consistent with a clinical practice sensitive to the parents' role and unconstrained either by an over-simplistic vitalism, excessive fear of legal liability or an emotionally appealing but ethically untenable distinction between withholding or withdrawing treatment. This strategy both re-cognizes and reflects the complex nature of these dilemmas. It is not without flaws—but it is probably the best that doctors, parents, and society can do.

The allocation of scarce resources

Questions about the routine or selective use of neonatal intensive care raise difficult dilemmas in the utilization of scarce resources, but doctors are uneasy about the need to make choices for patient care based on economics. As the costs of medical care escalate and shortages begin to affect patients, there are calls for increased spending on the National Health Service (NHS), on the one hand, and demands for more equitable distribution of resources, on the other. Few agree on priorities. Decisions on allocation inevitably raise questions that are as much ethical as medical and economic (Boyd and Potter 1986). If resources are finite and demands infinite it is inevitable that some form of rationing will result. At the present time kidney dialysis, intensive care, and coronary artery surgery are much less widely available in this country than in the USA (Schwartz and Aaron 1984).

The need to limit resources makes doctors very uncomfortable. While they are realistic enough to recognize that a 'blank cheque' is impossible, they insist that they must have freedom to do and spend whatever is necessary for their patients. They consider the 'common good' as secondary to the individual patient, a view that brings them into conflict with the new profession of health economists whose primary concern is to make maximum use of resources for the health of the community as a whole (Mooney 1984).

Doctors will 'ration' life-saving or life-prolonging treatments if they believe that they will be of no benefit to individual patients. There is the risk that this may become a form of rationalization to make economic decisions more acceptable. Patients (and parents) will vary in their willingness to accept passively that treatments will not be of benefit and some will be suspicious that they are being denied on economic grounds. We can expect to see competing demands for greater use of new technologies like kidney dialysis or transplantation and, at the same time, calls for a reduction in the waiting lists for psychogeriatric care or for such an effective operation as hip replacement. How can resources be allocated between these very different types of priority—doctors would certainly have one view, and I suspect that health economists would have another.

The use of scarce or expensive resources for one patient or group of patients inevitably will reduce the quality or quantity of care available to others. Perhaps it is the patients, the consumers, who eventually must decide on the priorities or at least be prepared to take more part in decisions. One aim of the new management structure in the NHS is to devolve budgets to clinical areas. As a result doctors may lose some of their control over what is spent on their wards, but if they remain totally aloof and refuse to cooperate in making more efficient decisions economically they may lose any ability to influence decisions on behalf of patients.

One area where the provision of resources has failed to keep pace with demand is in the new-born intensive care unit. At the level of *macro-allocation* (decisions about which services to provide to which groups), there is concern that this service to a relatively small number of infants is expanding at a rate detrimental to the allocation of resources to other services for children. Yet there are many reports which indicate the inadequate state of neonatal care in the country as a whole. Many units remain poorly staffed and rely on private charities for much of their basic equipment. If we consider the proportion of the gross national product spent on health in this country—compared with other developed countries—we must not spend time arguing about how the 'cake is sliced' but be seeking ways to increase the overall size of the 'cake' to help correct these inadequacies and inequalities.

At the same time it might be argued that, if difficult decisions have to be made, it surely makes sense and is morally more defensible to give priority to prevention rather than to the treatment of end-stage disease. Most activities within the field of child health are preventive yet child health, especially hospital paediatrics, has been given low priority in various funding formulae developed by DHSS and the Scottish Home and Health Department. Many have argued that skimping on the care of the new-born infants is false economy (Speidel 1986). It seems obvious, at least to paediatricians, that to prevent avoidable handicap through high quality neonatal care is not only a blessing for individual families but extremely cost-effective.

At the level of *micro-allocation* within neonatal units (choices about which individuals should benefit from the resources available) the indiscriminate or selective use of skills and technologies has already been discussed on the basis of what seems best for individual infants and families. Realistically it may also need to be considered in relation to available resources. Providing intensive care for all infants born alive whatever the birth-weight, gestational age, or condition may seriously affect the ability of an overloaded and understaffed unit to provide appropriate care for other infants, perhaps with serious consequences. Restricting the use of resources on medically sound quality-of-life criteria in the best interests of infants and families seems morally at least as defensible as refusing admission because the unit is full or withholding intermittent positive pressure ventilation because there are no more respirators. Like Jennett (1984) in his Rock Carling lecture on the inappropriate deployment of high technology medicine, neonatologists might ask themselves, for each case, if the treatments proposed are likely to be unsuccessful, unsafe, unkind, or unwise.

Telling the truth to parents and children

'The truth, the whole truth, and nothing but the truth' is well known in courts of law but is it a principle that must always be maintained in relationships with patients? There are times and situations when the stark truth about an operation or illness, no matter how sensitively presented, may be counter-productive to care and perhaps destructive of hope. There are differences of opinion about the extent to which a doctor must outline the risks of treatment when obtaining consent. As autonomy has replaced paternalism in decision-making, truth-telling is even more relevant to an adequately informed consent. The recent Sidaway decision in the House of Lords indicated that a doctor has a duty to warn of any *material* risk which might influence the patient in giving or withholding consent unless there are grounds (which should be sufficient to defend in court) to believe that such warnings might be detrimental to the patient's health (Brahams 1985). Inevitably much is left to clinical judgment, something that disturbs lawyers but is defended by doctors who feel that discretion is an essential element in dealing with the sometimes uniquely differing problems of individual patients. As with so many other ethical issues there is little place for the absolute rules that could result from unthinking application of a 'blunt instrument' like the law. Patients are people and all are different. Some will insist on knowing the whole truth and mean it; a few will not want to hear bad news, and the rest, perhaps the majority, will have enormously varying degrees of ambivalence. All this makes the judgment of truth-telling extremely difficult. Years of experience and 'long antennae' are needed to get it right even part of the time. Facts must be distinguished from speculation. Truth is important but confidence and trust in the doctor may be eroded either by repeated expressions of ignorance or by predictions and promises that have no hope of being realized.

When the patient is a child the arguments for honesty and complete openness with the parents are much more compelling. Parents need to be kept fully informed and up-to-date on details of diagnosis, treatment, and prognosis as far as they are known to the doctors. An understandable wish to shield one or both parents from the truth is usually a serious mistake and will undermine trust not only in the doctor but perhaps between parents. The overriding consideration must be the best interests of the child patient. Each child and each family must be considered individually in the context of the clinical facts in trying to work out how much or in what way the truth is told. What is told to the child will depend on the parents' and doctors' assessment of emotional maturity and level of understanding. Although the age of consent is 16 years in England and Wales (in Scotland, 12 years for girls and 14 years for boys) most children are able to give varying degrees of assent from 7 years onwards. However, telling all and giving too much detail will be largely incomprehensible and may be terrifying to a child already scared by the experience of being in hospital. In most circumstances it will be appropriate to withhold certain information from a child but it would be wrong to withhold *any* information about the child's condition from the parents. It has been argued, rightly in my view, that the degree of disclosure of the nature and risks of any proposed procedure is significantly different (i.e. should be greater) when a doctor advises parents about a child as opposed to advice given directly to a patient (Brahams 1986). In summary, therefore, 'The truth, the whole truth and nothing but the truth' is an important principle when talking to parents but we must adapt the words, the depth of detail, and the circumstances of the telling to the individual child's needs.

Confidentiality in under-16-year-olds

One of the most strongly held principles of medical ethics is that of confidentiality between a doctor and a patient, yet medical confidences (unlike legal) are not privileged in the law courts. Concern has been expressed that recent developments have undermined this principle (Havard 1984). In 1985 the General Medical Council (GMC), discussing advice on pregnancy and contraception, advised that if a doctor is not satisfied about a child's maturity and ability to understand the issues involved then he may inform the parents or person *in loco parentis*. The British Medical Association was reported to be 'deeply worried' by this ruling and insisted that a girl must have complete confidence in the confidentiality of the consultation. On the controversial case that stimulated this debate the House of Lords finally decided (by a majority) that doctors can treat children provided that the child has been properly informed and understands what is involved (Dyer 1985).

Almost certainly paediatricians, like others, will have very different views on this issue. However, paediatricians, more than most, will be aware of the great variation in physical, psychological, and emotional development in girls during their adolescent years. These differences, together with variations in intelligence and education, make it illogical and undesirable to use age as the only criterion for deciding to provide advice on such important matters as contraception and termination of pregnancy with or without parental knowledge or consent. Paediatricians are also aware of the importance of family life and parental responsibility in bringing up children. This responsibility will include guidance on sexual matters, usually assumed by mothers, so that a girl develops a gradual understanding of the implications of sexual relationships, contraception, pregnancy, and abortion. Unfortunately, and for a variety of reasons, some girls will not get this help or will have become sufficiently alienated from parents to make them seek help, if they seek help at all, from the family doctor or a doctor at a Family Planning Clinic. There must be some room for discretion in these extremely difficult and sad situations and the GMC's advice properly took account of this need for discretion and the use of clinical judgment.

In most situations doctors will seek the girl's permission to contact the parents or urge the girl to inform her parents herself, but if permission is refused the doctor must keep the details of the consultation in the strictest confidence and be prepared to provide advice and treatment without parental knowledge. 'Those who read the full report of the judgment ... cannot fail to appreciate the importance of the ruling for the future, for it means that absolute parental authority has gone' (Editorial 1986). Nevertheless Lord Fraser in giving the judgement referred to above warned doctors not to disregard the wishes of parents whenever they find it convenient to do so. Certainly there will be exceptional circumstances but these must be documented carefully. There will be times when it will be 'right' to inform the parents in the best interests of the child just as there will be times when it will be 'right' to prevent an unwanted pregnancy without reference to parents. Sadly, the fact that so many young girls now consult a doctor without parental knowledge is some reflection of how badly communication has broken down within families. This recent House of Lords ruling places additional responsibilities on doctors but if they use and are seen to use their discretionary powers wisely for the benefit of the child while working as closely as possible with the parents their reward may include the restoration of contact and trust between a girl and her family.

In-vitro fertilization and embryo research

Alternative methods of reproduction   Infertility is the cause of much heartache and affects about 1 in 10 couples. There are many causes.

Some treatments pose few ethical dilemmas but are likely to help only a few infertile couples. Recent developments of donor insemination, *in-vitro* fertilization (IVF), surrogate parenting, and embryo transfer raise profound ethical issues, but calm and careful consideration and agreement on the moral issues raised by these developments have lagged behind the technical advances. Perhaps most importantly for paediatricians, little attention has been paid to the implications for the products of these techniques, the children themselves (Sokoloff 1987). The complexities are considerable. For example, it is now possible for a child to have five 'parents': a genetic and a rearing father, and a genetic, a gestational, and a rearing mother. There are also major implications for the family as a social unit and for the future fabric of our society, so that paediatricians as advocates for children need assurance that the emotional and psychological health of the participants are also being considered. Concern about confidentiality has been, and will remain, a major difficulty in addressing these issues, but as the techniques become refined and gain public acceptance much of the current ignorance and stigmatization should disappear. It is particularly important that epidemiological mechanisms are developed that will identify problems that may arise among these 'high-risk children'.

Most paediatricians probably are in broad agreement with the recommendations outlined in the Warnock Report (1978) and welcome these new treatments for infertility provided that appropriate methods of surveillance and control are developed to prevent abuse. At the time of writing the Department of Health and Social Security (DHSS 1986) has issued a consultation paper on the form that legislation might take to control human infertility services and embryo research.

There are a number of issues that particularly concern paediatricians:

1. If a Statutory Licensing Authority (SLA) is established its membership should include a children's physician.

2. The interests of the child conceived by these techniques should be paramount. Problems relating to the care and nurture of the children after birth should receive as much attention as the problems of conception and embryo culture. Legislation must be protective of all the members of the infertile family, and the child conceived by these techniques must not be disadvantaged but given equal

status to other children. Legal rights should continue to be assured in the event of divorce or death of the parents.

3. The licensing of these techniques should require the availability of adequate counselling for the potential parents. Training programmes for counsellors should be established, and experience gained by the adoption services over many years utilised in protecting the best interests of the children.

4. In addition to counselling the infertile couple it will be important to have appropriate medical screening prior to any decision on eligibility.

5. There is continuing debate about the medical, moral, and legal justification for extending these techniques to single women and lesbians. This arouses strong feelings, and calm consideration of responsibilities and duties to the future child becomes difficult in the face of strident demands for individual 'rights'. In thinking primarily about the interests of the child it must be asked if his or her future under such an arrangement might be too uncertain to justify his or her creation? Are we worried that raising a child in the absence of a father is in the best interests of that child even accepting that many single parents, through necessity, have successfully raised many fine children? Because of our continuing belief in the two-parent family as a desirable social unit perhaps these techniques should be restricted to conventional married couples or similar stable relationships.

6. Complete anonymity of donors must be assured but some linkage system of non-identifying information must be maintained, perhaps by the Registrar General, to allow important epidemiological study of these families and the future progress of the children.

7. There is considerable anxiety about the implications of surrogacy. Most paediatricians would agree with the legislation to ban commercial surrogacy under the Surrogacy Arrangements Act 1985, although they are perhaps surprised that the commissioning parents and the surrogate mother cannot be held liable. The status of non-commercial surrogacy remains confused. Surrogacy of any kind is a potential medical, moral, and legal minefield in which widespread concern about the psychological and emotional effects on the adult participants so far has diverted proper attention from the implications for the child. The recent legislation concentrated on the commissioning parents and the surrogate mother but the

real issue that must be faced by the courts now and in the future is what must be done to protect the interests of the child.

Embryo research

Embryo research offers exciting prospects for reducing the incidence of congenital abnormalities and resulting handicap. Screening high-risk embryos before implantation and treating genetic disorders should bring great benefits to individual families. Perhaps more than most, paediatricians are aware of the devastating effects that some congenital abnormalities can have on individual children and their families and would support such research wholeheartedly. Some might argue that our enhanced ability to ensure the birth of only 'perfect' children has already led to an intolerance of imperfection which would be further enhanced by genetic manipulation. Surely the tragedy of birth abnormality makes the aim of ultimate elimination of all birth defects almost a moral imperative? Why should parents not hope for a 'perfect child'? If this could be a result of this new technology we should strive to achieve it.

Although it is not possible at present to keep embryos alive for more than a few days it is inevitable that future developments will achieve much longer *in vitro* survival. The current restriction of 14 days proposed in the Warnock Report is a reasonable 'first step', but it will become restrictive as technology advances. If maximum benefit is to be achieved by embryo research it may be prudent and equally defensible morally to extend the limit to six weeks, the time when developments in the central nervous system suggest that this may be when the embryo first develops a sense of awareness. (Council for Science and Society 1984.)

Another aspect that should concern paediatricians is whether research should be confined to 'spare embryos' or could be extended to embryos created purely for research purposes. As IVF becomes more efficient the number of spare embryos is likely to decline and important genetic research might be inhibited. Embryo research of any kind is abhorrent to many people who would argue that 'human beings' should never be used as means to an end but be respected as ends in themselves. Others see no moral distinction between the use of embryos available as by-products of IVF and those deliberately created for research and believe that such research should be allowed provided it is subject to appropriate surveillance.

Embryo research offers great promise to future generations. It would be sad if appropriately authorized research were to be inhibited either by being restricted to 14 days or by making illegal the creation of embryos for research. It has been argued that 'it would be quixotic (and irresponsible) to ban such research on the basis of moral arguments which are inadequately worked out'; and to be consistent we should also ban most of the abortions permitted by contemporary abortion legislation (Brown 1986).

Whether or not families decide to seek help for infertility and participate in these new techniques should remain a matter of individual choice. Legislation should be limited to the control of standards and the prevention of abuses through either a Voluntary Licensing Authority as at present or the Statutory Licensing Authority proposed in the Warnock Report.

Children as subjects of medical research

Research has been and is of great importance to children past, present, and future. Nevertheless paediatricians and other investigators continue to face troubling questions of conscience in designing and carrying out research or find that even proposals which they consider to be above reproach do not receive the approval of a local ethics advisory committee. The main stumbling block to universal acceptance of using children as research subjects remains the problem of voluntary consent, impossible to obtain in the young. There is also continuing uncertainty about the legal basis of parental or proxy consent especially for *non-therapeutic research*, although it is generally accepted that parents may give permission for a child to take part in research that is part of necessary treatment and therefore for the child's benefit, i.e. *therapeutic research*. Still widely quoted is an interpretation of the law given to the Medical Research Council (MRC) and incorporated in its 1963 guidelines: ' . . . in the strict view of the law, parents and guardians of minors cannot give consent on their behalf to any procedures which are of no particular benefit to them and which may cause some risk of harm'. At that time, it must be remembered, there was growing professional and public alarm about reports condemning some of the research being conducted in reputable and often distinguished medical centres where informed consent was seen to be inadequate and the trust implicit in the doctor–patient relationship had been abused however unwittingly (Beecher 1966; Pappworth 1967).

It seemed obvious that some tightening of controls was necessary. Indeed, during the 1950s and early 1960s much less control was exerted over research with human subjects than with animals. Guidelines were needed which would allow important research to continue yet provide adequate protection for the individual experimental subjects. Children were recognized to be particularly vulnerable to exploitation by unscrupulous researchers but because of strict interpretation of the MRC guidelines it seemed possible that their participation, even in valuable research, might have to cease altogether. In 1973 a Royal College of Physicians report entitled *Supervision of the ethics of clinical research investigations in institutions* recognized the potential seriousness of this situation when it stated:

If advances in medical treatment are to continue so must clinical research investigation. It is in this light therefore that it is recommended that clinical research investigation of children or mentally handicapped adults which is not of direct benefit to the patient should be conducted, but only when the procedures entail negligible risk or discomfort and subject to the provision of any common and statute law prevailing at the time. The parent or guardian should be consulted and his agreement recorded.

In spite of this encouragement from such a prestigious institution, uncertainty about the legal position remained, and a statement by the Chief Medical Officer (DHSS) of the time did not help to reassure investigators: 'It is not legitimate to perform any experiment on a child that is not in the child's interests' (Godber 1974).

It has been pointed out that the MRC statement was based on one, but only one, legal opinion and did not have any basis in statute or in case law (Curran and Beecher 1969; Campbell 1974; Dworkin 1978). There never has been a test case. Moreover, careful reading of the MRC (1963) document also indicated that lack of benefit from the research was coupled with risk of harm. Thus a strictly utilitarian costs/benefits analysis might be applied to human research and it seemed possible that even some paediatric research could be justified if the parents gave permission, if the benefits clearly outweighed the risks, and if the research had received the approval of an ethics advisory committee, a number of which were then being established in most health districts or areas. In his extensive review of the topic Beecher (1970) believed it to be:

. . . tenable and reasonable to consider that parents have the right to decide whether their children will participate in experimentation even if not for their direct benefit, provided the studies contemplated have no discernable risk and have been approved by a high-level review committee as necessary and valuable for human progress and do not unfairly take advantage of the child.

The BPA Working Party on ethical aspects of paediatric research began its report by stating four basic premises:

1. That research involving children is important for the benefit of all children and should be supported and encouraged, and conducted in an ethical manner.
2. That research should never be done on children if the same investigation could be done on adults.
3. That research which involves a child and is of no benefit to that child (non-therapeutic research) is not necessarily either unethical or illegal.
4. That the degree of benefit resulting from a research should be assessed in relation to the risk of disturbance, discomfort or pain—the 'Risk/Benefit ratio' (British Paediatric Association 1980).

The Working Party went on to define what they meant by 'risk' and 'benefit' and indicated how the risk/benefit principle could be applied to therapeutic and non-therapeutic research. Less attention was paid to the problem of proxy consent. The report merely contained a statement indicating that 'Parental (or Guardian's) permission should *normally* (my italics) be obtained . . . after explaining as fully as possible the nature of the procedure'. The suggestion that 'It is an advantage if the parents can be present during the procedure' could be seen as another way in which the group were anxious to strengthen the protection of the child.

Commendably brief and clearly expressed, these guidelines were welcomed by investigators anxious to have authoritative guidance in planning research and looking for support in discussions with ethics committees. A number of statements in the report have been questioned in a recent book (Nicholson 1986), but while some issues would benefit from further clarification and revision, its balanced, common-sense, and sensitive approach remains as valid today as it was in 1980.

In the USA the National Commission for the Protection of Human Subjects of Biomedical and Behavioural Research established by Congress in 1974 was also paying particular attention to the problems of proxy consent and risk/benefit assessment. After a prolonged gestation period for consultation the final Federal regulations were issued in 1983 (US Department of Health and Human Services 1983). Four categories of research involving risk/benefit criteria were considered:

1. Research not involving greater than minimal risk.
2. Research involving greater than minimal risk but presenting the prospect of direct benefit to individual subjects.
3. Research involving greater than minimal risk and no prospect of direct benefit to individual subjects, but likely to yield generalised knowledge about the subject's disorder or condition.
4. Research not otherwise approvable which presents an opportunity to understand, prevent or alleviate a serious problem affecting the health or welfare of children.

The US regulations place more emphasis and additional responsibilities on Institutional Review Boards (IRBs), the rough equivalent of British Ethics Advisory Committees. They require IRBs to determine for each project:
1. If it is scientifically sound and significant.
2. If it was first performed on animals and adults and then in older children.
3. If the risks are minimized by using the safest procedures consistent with research design.
4. If privacy and confidentiality are to be respected.
5. If the subjects are to be selected in an equitable manner.
6. If the diagnostic and therapeutic procedures are standard.
7. If there has been permission of parents and the assent of children when capable.

The Commission considered that research which does not involve greater than minimal risk could be conducted provided that the above conditions are met. It is always difficult to find definitions that please everyone but the definition of 'minimal' as 'The probability and magnitude of physical and psychological harm that is usually encountered in the daily lives or in the routine medical or psychological examination of healthy children' is very similar to that proposed by the BPA Working Group and makes sense to most people. Examples would be immunization, dietary changes, developmental assessments, and blood and urine tests. The Commission pointed out that disruption of normal routine and the effects of separation from parents should not be forgotten.

For risks *greater than minimal* the Commission approved of *therapeutic* research provided the ratio of anticipated benefit to risk was at least as favourable as other treatment alternatives including that of no treatment.

For *non-therapeutic* research with *greater than minimal* risk strong differences of opinion emerged among members of the Commission. By a majority (there were two dissenting voices) it was decided that an absolute prohibition was unreasonable. The Commission quoted the example of children with rare diseases who are the only sources of information about these conditions and where results of studies may bring great benefit to succeeding sufferers. It listed some criteria to help decide when children may participate in such research:

a. The risk is a minor increase over minimal risk.
b. The procedures or tests performed are already something within the experience of the child as part of its treatment, e.g. a biopsy or a lumbar puncture.
c. The research is likely to yield knowledge of vital importance for understanding and for ameliorating the condition from which the subject suffers.

Thus after prolonged and careful analysis of the issues, the US Commission and the BPA Working Party appeared to accept that both therapeutic *and* non-therapeutic research with children may be justifiable ethically on the basis of a utilitarian cost–benefit analysis with the permission of the parents and with approval of an ethics advisory committee. This is also the conclusion of the Working Party set up recently by the Institute of Medical Ethics. It seems that all these groups accept that the primacy of the research subject need not always be considered paramount, but in certain circumstances his or her interests may be seen as secondary to the interests of others or society. As adults we have a moral responsibility to help others in society and we should instil this sense of responsibility in our children. Beecher (1970) implied as much in his introduction to the problems of research in children:

Parents have the obligation to inculcate into their children attitudes of unselfish service. One would hope that this might be extended to include participation in research for the public welfare when it is important and there is no discernible risk.

Gaylin (1982) makes the same point in an amusing story about a friend who took his 10-year-old son for a physical examination:

The doctor having completed the examination, turned to the child formally and asked permission to take a small sample of blood for an epidemiological study that he was doing on a major childhood disease. As the father related the story, the doctor, in a somewhat precious way, explained to the child that this was not part of his examination but would help some other little boys. Johnny asked the doctor 'Will it hurt'? The doctor answered 'a little—like a pinprick'. Johnny said 'I don't want it', whereupon the father said to his son 'Listen young man, you just get your hand up on that table and let the doctor take the blood'. Johnny, recognising the note of authority in the father's voice immediately complied whereupon the doctor, forgetting the formalism of his original consent proceedings gladly took the sample. In explaining the situation to me the father said that his reaction was not just an expression of authoritarianism or paternalism; he had a moral obligation to teach his child that there are certain things one does even if they cause a small amount of pain, to benefit others. 'I was less concerned with the research involved than with the kind of boy I was raising'.

Recently it has been argued that non-therapeutic research may be justified on deontological grounds if we can reasonably expect that, like the parents who gave consent, the child in later life would identify with the objects of the research and believe it to be worthwhile (Redmon 1986). In the UK the supervising arrangements, i.e. Ethics Advisory Committees, are too inconsistent in constitution and responsibility. Their responses to similar research proposals show great variations from region to region. Ethics Committees will need to be constituted rather differently if they are to carry out their responsibilities properly. The Institute of Medical Ethics Working Group suggests *inter alia* that it is time to make them legally based. I agree that they do need to be strengthened and their membership made more consistent. They must also be given more authority, for example, to require the mandatory submission of all projects, but I hope that 'legal' involvement can be restricted to giving them appropriate authority vested in their local health authority or governing body. Many doctors and lawyers feel that to otherwise involve the law in delineating the boundaries of research and perhaps prohibiting some research on children would be clumsy and unwise and represent an unwarranted intrusion between parent and child. The law remains to be tested, and with adequate professional controls it should remain untested. We must ensure that controls not only are adequate but are seen to be adequate. Parental consent must remain the key item in these controls. Recently controversy has erupted over the practice of entering newly born infants in research studies without the consent or even knowledge of their parents. This practice has been defended by some neonatologists who point out the great practical difficulties as well as the excessive anxiety likely to be engendered by such a discussion at the time of birth. Much of this research can be defined as 'therapeutic' and will include studies using random allocation to one or more standard treatments or to a new treatment. In this country it is undoubtedly carried out by investigators of integrity, which in itself provides some protection, but I think most of the public would view lack of parental awareness or permission as highly undesirable if not unacceptable.

About 40 years ago a distinguished honorary member of the BPA wrote

It is still more difficult to approach a newly delivered mother about an experiment on her baby, even if this only involves a study of how it breathes, and the inclination to make the experiment without doing so is very great. Patients and parents, however, rarely refuse and in my experience opposition to experimental work in hospital generally comes from colleagues under whom the patients have been admitted and from the nursing staff who are, in general, antagonistic to research, especially on children (McCance 1950).

It is absolutely vital that controlled trials are allowed or history will continue to record the disastrous consequences of introducing new therapies uncritically (Silverman 1985). Parents are usually aware of the benefits to be derived from skills and facilities available in large hospitals where most of this research is conducted. They should be made aware of current research and its importance. In many instances approval of the research and permission for infants to participate, if appropriate, could be obtained prenatally. Explanatory leaflets about research could become available as part of routine antenatal care. This would of course not absolve investigators from further detailed and specific discussion with confirmation of the consent at a suitable time after birth, but at least it would allow them to enter infants in their studies immediately without fear of moral opprobrium or legal action. We must create a climate of opinion where research under proper safeguards is seen to be an appropriate, even essential, part of caring for children.

Appendix I: Ethics of research

The Nuremberg Code (1947)

The protagonists of the practice of human experimentation justify their views on the basis that such experiments yield results for the good of society that are improcurable by other methods or means of study. All agree however, that certain basic principles must be observed in order to satisfy moral, ethical and legal concepts:

1. The voluntary consent of the human subject is absolutely essential. This means that the person involved should have legal capacity to give consent; should be so situated as to be able to exercise free power of choice; without the intervention of any element of force, fraud, deceit, duress, over-reaching, or other ulterior form of constraint or coercion; and should have sufficient knowledge and comprehension of the elements of the subject matter involved as to enable him to make an understanding and enlightened decision.

World Medical Association: Declaration of Geneva (1948)

I solemnly pledge myself to consecrate my life to the service of humanity.
I will practice my profession with conscience and dignity.
The health of my patient will be my first consideration;
I will respect the secrets which are confided in me;
I will maintain by all the means in my power, the honour and noble traditions of the medical profession;
I will not permit considerations of religion, nationality, race, party politics or social standing to intervene between my duty and my patient;
I will maintain the utmost respect for human life from the time of conception; even under threat, I will not use my medical knowledge contrary to the laws of humanity.

Medical Research Council: responsibility in investigation on human subjects (1963)

Investigations that are of no direct benefit to the individual require therefore that his true consent to them shall be explicitly obtained . . .

When the subject is below the age of 12 years information regarding the performance of any procedure involving his body would need to be obtained incidentally to and without altering the nature of a procedure intended for his individual benefit.

. . . in the strict view of the law, parents or guardians of minors cannot give consent on their behalf to any procedures which are of no particular benefit to them and which may carry some risk of harm.

Royal College of Physicians of London: supervision of the ethics of clinical research investigations in institutions (1973)

If advances in medical treatment are to continue so must clinical research investigation. It is in this light therefore that it is recommended that clinical research investigation of children or mentally handicapped adults which is not of direct benefit to the patient should be conducted ... but only when the procedures entail negligible risk or discomfort and subject to the provisions of any common or statute law prevailing at the time. The parent or guardian should be consulted and his agreement recorded.

World Medical Association: Declaration of Helsinki (1964, revised 1975)

In the field of biomedical research a fundamental distinction must be recognised between medical research in which the aim is essentially diagnostic or therapeutic for a patient, and medical research, the essential object of which is purely scientific, and without direct diagnostic or therapeutic value to the person subjected to the research.

In case of legal incompetence, informed consent should be obtained from the legal guardian in accordance with national legislation. Where physical or mental incapacity makes it impossible to obtain informed consent, or when the subject is a minor, permission from the responsible relative replaces that of the subject in accordance with national legislation.

British Paediatric Association: guidelines to aid ethical committees considering research involving children (1980)

Research involving children is important for the benefit of all children and should be supported and encouraged, and conducted in an ethical manner.

Research should never be done on children if the same investigations could be done on adults.

Research which involves the child and is of no benefit to that child (non-therapeutic research), is not necessarily either unethical or illegal. The degree of benefit resulting from a research should be assessed in relation to the risk of disturbance, discomfort, or pain—the 'Risk/Benefit' ratio . . .

. . . Parental (or guardian's) permission should normally be obtained— with rare exceptions such as the comparison of two treatments for some emergency condition—after explaining as fully as possible the nature of the procedure. Whether or not this should be a signed witnessed declaration remains debatable. It is an advantage if the parents can be present during the procedure. Although the law in Britain does not recognise an 'age of consent', children much younger than 16 often have enough understanding to collaborate altruistically in a project.

Institute of Medical Ethics: medical research with children: ethics, law and practice (1986)

Recommendations of Working Group
General conclusions:
We recommend that:

. . . research requiring children as subjects should not be undertaken unless there is a specific and demonstrable need to perform the research on children, and no other route to the relevant knowledge is available.

. . . further efforts be made to develop scales quantifying risk and benefit, so as to reduce reliance on the qualitative descriptions of risk in use at present.

. . . non-therapeutic research procedures should not be carried out, if they involve greater than minimal risk to any individual child subject.

. . . there should be a limit on the number of times that an innovative therapy may be used on children, without its being submitted as a formal research project to a research ethics committee.

Parents and children:
We recommend that:

. . . parents and guardians should be considered as trustees of a child's interests, rather than as having rights over the child. The prime consideration in any research involving children should be that it be not against the interest of any individual child.

. . . proxy consent by parents or guardians to a non-therapeutic research procedure on their child is legally valid and ethically acceptable only when the risk of such research to the child subject is no more than minimal.

   1. for consent to be valid on all (or any) interpretations of existing law, the consent of parent or guardian be required at all ages of the child;

furthermore, the child's assent should be sought from the age of 7 upwards.

2. on a cautious view of the law, consent be deemed not to have been given if the parent or guardian of a child below 16 years refuses consent, *or* if a child over 14 years refuses consent.

3. notwithstanding the desirability of seeking the child's assent, for a child aged 7 to 14 years, the decision of parent or guardian to give consent for a therapeutic research procedure be deemed to override the refusal of assent by the child.

4. a non-therapeutic research procedure should not be carried out if a potential child subject aged 7 to 14 years refuses assent to it.

Investigators:

We recommend that:

. . . all proposals for research on children be submitted to the appropriate research ethics committee for consideration.

. . . investigators be encouraged to recognise that the research enterprise should be a partnership *with* the child subjects and their parents or guardians, rather than an activity undertaken *on* children.

. . . in assessing the risks of a research project to an individual child subject investigators take account not only of the risks of any proposed research procedures but also of the cumulative medical, emotional, and social risks to which the child is already exposed or may become exposed, whether or not as a consequence of the research interventions.

Appendix II: severely disabled infants

Guidelines on the care of severely malformed infants (agreed by the Ethics Advisory Committees of the British Paediatric Association and the British Medical Association (1983)

A malformed infant has the same rights as a normal infant. It follows that ordinary non-medical care which is necessary for the maintenance of the life of a normal infant should not be withheld from a malformed infant.

Where medical or surgical measures might be needed to preserve the life of a severely malformed infant, every opportunity should be taken for deliberation and discussion, as time permits. This requires the closest cooperation between the doctor in charge, the parents of the child, and any colleagues whose opinion is felt to be helpful, including the patient's general practitioner. The doctors have a particular duty to ensure that parents have as full an understanding as possible of the options and the likely outcome, with or without surgery or other means of active intervention.

The parents of an infant born severely malformed must never be left with the feeling that they are having to exercise their responsibility to make decisions regarding consent to the management of their child without help and understanding. They should be encouraged to seek advice from anyone in whose judgment they have faith. The doctor in charge is responsible for the initiation or the withholding of treatment in the best interests of the infant. He must attend primarily to the needs and rights of the individual infant, and he must also have concern for the family as a whole. If doubts persist in the minds either of the parents or doctor in charge as to the best interests of the infant a second medical opinion should be sought.

In emergencies there may be no time for consultation with parents or anyone else, and the doctor in charge must exercise his clinical judgment.

US President's commission for the study of ethical problems in medicine and biomedical and behavioural research: deciding to forego life-sustaining treatment (*1983*)

Seriously ill newborns.

13. Parents should be the surrogates for a seriously ill newborn unless they are disqualified by decision-making incapacity, an unresolvable disagreement between them, or their choice of a course of action that is clearly against the infant's best interests.

14. Therapies expected to be futile for a seriously ill newborn need not be provided; parents, health care professionals and institutions, and reimbursement sources however should ensure the infant's comfort.

15. Within constraints of equity and availability, infants should receive all therapies that are clearly beneficial to them. For example, an otherwise healthy Down's Syndrome child whose life is threatened by a surgically correctable complication should receive the surgery because he or she would clearly benefit from it.

    (a) The concept of benefit necessarily makes reference to the context of the infant's present and future treatment, taking into account such matters as the level of biomedical knowledge and technology, and the availability of services necessary for the child's treatment.

    (b) The dependence of benefit upon context underlines society's special obligation to provide necessary services for handicapped children and their families, which rests on the special ethical duties owed to newborns with undeserved disadvantages and on the general ethical duty of the community to ensure equitable access for all persons to an adequate level of health care.

16. Decision-makers should have access to the most accurate and up-to-date information as they consider individual cases.

    (a) Physicians should obtain appropriate consultation and referrals.

(b) The significance of the diagnoses and the prognoses under each treatment option must be conveyed to the parents (or other surrogates).

17. The medical staff, administrators, and trustees of each institution that provides care to seriously ill newborns should take the responsibility for ensuring good decision-making practices. Accrediting bodies may want to require that institutions have appropriate policies in this area.

(a) An institution should have clear and explicit policies that require prospective or retrospective review of decisions when life-sustaining treatment for an infant might be foregone or when parents and providers disagree about the correct decision for an infant. Certain categories of clearly futile therapies could be explicitly excluded from review.

(b) The best interests of an infant should be pursued when those interests are clear.

(c) The policies should allow for the exercise of parental discretion when a child's interests are ambiguous.

(d) Decisions should be referred to public agencies (including courts) for review when necessary to determine whether parents should be disqualified as decision-makers and, if so, who should decide the course of treatment that would be in the best interests of their child.

American Academy of Paediatrics: principles of treatment of disabled infants (1984)

When medical care is clearly beneficial, it should always be provided. When appropriate medical care is not available, arrangements should be made to transfer the infant to an appropriate medical facility. Considerations such as an anticipated or actual limited potential of an individual, and present or future lack of available community resources are irrelevant and must not determine the decisions concerning medical care. The individual's medical condition should be the sole focus of the decision. These are very strict standards.

American Medical Association: policy statement (1984)

Quality of Life. In the making of decisions for the treatment of seriously deformed newborns or persons who are seriously deteriorated victims of injury, illness or advanced age, the primary consideration should be what is best for the individual patients and not the avoidance of a burden to the family or to society. Quality of life is a factor to be considered in determining what is best for the individual. Life should be cherished despite disabilities and handicaps, except when prolongation would be inhumane and unconscionable. Under these circumstances, withholding or removing life supporting means is ethical provided that the normal care given an individual who is ill is not discontinued.

In desperate situations involving newborns the advice and judgment of the physicians should be readily available but the decision whether to exert maximal efforts to sustain life should be the choice of the parents. The parents should be told the options, expected benefits, risks and limits of any proposed care; how the potential for human relationships is affected by the infant's condition; and relevant information and answers to their questions. The presumption is that the love which parents usually have for their children will be dominant in the decision which they make in determining what is in the best interest of their children. It is to be expected that parents will act unselfishly, particularly where life itself is at stake. Unless there is convincing evidence to the contrary, parental authority should be respected.

References

Angell, M. (1983). Handicapped children: Baby Doe and Uncle Sam. *New England Journal of Medicine* **309**, pp. 659-61.

Beecher, H. K. (1966), Ethics and clinical research. *New England Journal of Medicine* **274**, pp. 1354-60.

Beecher, H. K. (1970), *Research and the individual: human studies* Little, Brown, Boston, MA.

Boyd, K. M. and Potter, B. T. (1986). Priorities in the allocation of scarce resources. *Journal of Medical Ethics* **12**, pp. 197-200.

Brahams, D. (1985). Doctor's duty to inform patients of substantial or special risks when offering treatment. *Lancet* **1**, pp. 528-30.

Brahams, D. (1986). Explanation and disclosure of risks in the treatment of children. *Lancet* **1**, pp. 925-6.

Brahams, D. and Brahams, M. (1983). The Arthur case—a proposal for legislation. *Journal of Medical Ethics* **9**, pp. 12-15.

British Paediatric Association (1980). Guidelines to aid ethical committees considering research involving children. *Archives of Disease in Childhood* **55**, pp. 75-7.

Brown, J. (1986). Research on human embryos—a justification. *Journal of Medical Ethics* **12**, pp. 201-5.

Budin, P. (1907). The nursling: the feeding and hygiene of premature and full-term infants. Caxton, London.

Campbell, A. G. M. (1974). Infants, children and informed consent. *British Medical Journal* **3**, pp. 334-8.

Campbell, A. G. M. (1982). Which infants should not receive intensive care? *Archives of Disease in Childhood* **57**, pp. 569-71.

Council for Science and Society (1984). *Human procreation: ethical aspects of the new techniques.* Report of the Working Party. Chairman: G. R. Dunstan. Oxford University Press, Oxford.

Curran, W. J. and Beecher, H. K. (1969). Experimentation in children: a re-examination of legal ethical principles. *Journal of the American Medical Association* **210**, pp. 77-83.

DHSS (1986). Legislation on human infertility services and embryo research. A consultation paper. Department of Health and Social Security. HMSO, London.

Duff, R. S. and Campbell, A. G. M. (1973). Moral and ethical dilemmas in the special-care nursery. *New England Journal of Medicine* **289**, pp. 890-4.

Duff, R. S. and Campbell, A. G. M. (1976). On deciding the care of severely handicapped or dying persons: with particular reference to infants. *Pediatrics* **57**, pp. 487-93.

Dworkin, G. (1978). Legality of consent to non-therapeutic medical research on infants and young children. *Archives of Disease in Childhood* **53**, pp. 443-6.

Dyer, C. (1985). Contraceptives and the under sixteens: House of Lords ruling. *British Medical Journal* **291**, pp. 1208-9.

Editorial (1986). *Archives of Disease in Childhood* **61**, pp. 725-6.

Etziony, M. B. (1973). *The physicians's creed*. Charles C Thomas, Springfield, IL.

Fleischman, A. R. (1986). An infant bioethical review committee in an urban medical center. *Hastings Center Report* **16**(3), pp. 16-18.

Forrest, D. M. (1967). Modern trends in the treatment of spina bifida: early closure in spina bifida: results and problems. *Proceedings of the Royal Society of Medicine* **60**, pp. 763-7.

Franklin, A. W. (1963). Physically handicapped babies: some thalidomide lessons. *Lancet* **1**, pp. 959-62.

Gaylin, W. (1982). The competence of children: no longer all or none. *Hastings Center Report* **12**(2), pp. 33-8.

Godber, G. (1974). Constraints upon the application of medical advances. *Proceedings of Royal Society of Medicine* **67**, p. 1311.

Havard, J. D. J. (1984). Protecting confidentiality. *British Medical Journal* **288**, pp. 1102-3.

Illingworth, R. S. and Illingworth, C. M. (1965). Thou shalt not kill: should thou strive to keep alive? *Clinical Pediatrics* **4**, pp. 305-8.

Jennett, B. (1984). *High technology medicine. Nuffield Provincial Hospital Trust*, London.

Ladd, J. (1980). Medical ethics: who knows best? *Lancet* **2**, pp. 1127-9.

Lorber, J. (1971). Results of treatment of meningomyelocele: an analysis of 524 unselected cases with special reference to possible selection for treatment. *Developmental Medicine and Child Neurology* **13**, pp. 279-303.

McCance, R. A. (1950). The practice of experimental medicine. *Proceedings of the Royal Society of Medicine* **44**, pp. 189-94.

Mooney, G. (1984). Medical ethics: an excuse for inefficiency? *Journal of Medical Ethics* **10**, pp. 183-5.

Nicholson, R. H. (1986). *Medical research with children: ethics, law and practice.* Oxford University Press, Oxford.

Pappworth, M. H. (1967). *Human guinea pigs.* Routledge and Kegan Paul, Andover, Hants.

Rachels, J. (1986). *The end of life: euthanasia and morality.* Oxford University Press, Oxford.

Redmon, R. B. (1986). How children can be respected as 'ends' yet still be used as subjects in non-therapeutic research. *Journal of Medical Ethics* **12**, pp. 77–82.

Rhoden, N. K. (1986). Treating Baby Doe: the ethics of uncertainty. *Hastings Center Report* **16**(4), pp. 34–42.

Robertson, J. A. and Fost, N. (1976). Passive euthanasia of defective newborn infants: legal considerations. *Journal of Pediatrics* **88**, pp. 883–9.

Schwartz, W. B. and Aaron, H. J. (1984). Rationing hospital care: lessons from Britain. *New England Journal of Medicine* **310**, pp. 52–6.

Shaw, A. (1973). Dilemmas of 'informed consent' in children. *New England Journal of Medicine* **289**, pp. 885–90.

Silverman, W. A. (1981). Mismatched attitudes about neonatal death. *Hastings Center Report* **11**(6), pp. 12–16.

Silverman, W. A. (1985). *Human experimentation: a guided step into the unknown.* Oxford University Press, Oxford.

Slater, E. (1971). Health service or sickness service. *Lancet* **2**, pp. 734–6.

Sokoloff, B. Z. (1987). Alternative methods of reproduction. *Clinical Pediatrics* **26**, pp. 11–17.

Speidel, B. D. (1986). Skimping on care of the newborn is false economy. *British Medical Journal* **293**, p. 575.

US Department of Health and Human Services (1983). Additional protections for children involved as subjects in research. *Federal Register* **48**, pp. 9814–20.

Warnock Report (1978). Special educational needs: report of the Committee of Enquiry into the Education of Handicapped Children and Young People. Chairwoman: H. M. Warnock, Cmnd 7212. HMSO, London.

Further Reading

Beauchamp, T. L. and Childress, J. F. (1983). *Principles of biomedical ethics* (2nd edn). Oxford University Press, Oxford.

Campbell, A. V. (1984). *Moral dilemmas in medicine: a casebook in ethics for doctors and nurses* (3rd edn). Churchill Livingstone, Edinburgh.

Goldstein, J., Freud, A., and Solnit, A. J. (1973). *Beyond the best interests of the child.* Collier Macmillan, West Drayton, Middx.

Goldstein, J., Freud, A., and Solnit, A. J. (1979), *Before the best interests of the child.* Collier Macmillan, West Drayton, Middx.

Guillemin, J. H. and Holmstrom, L. L. (1986). *Mixed blessings: intensive care for newborns.* Oxford University Press, Oxford.

Gustaitis, R. and Young, E. W. D. (1986). *A time to be born, a time to die: conflicts and ethics in an intensive care nursery*. Addison-Wesley, Reading, MA.

Keyserlingk, E. W. (1979). *Sanctity of life or quality of life in the context of ethics, medicine and law*. Law Reform Commission of Canada, Ottawa.

Kuhse, H. and Singer, P. (1985). *Should the baby live? The problem of handicapped infants*. Oxford University Press, Oxford.

Ladd, J. (ed.) (1979). *Ethical issues relating to life and death*. Oxford University Press, Oxford.

Linacre Centre (1982). *Euthanasia and clinical practice: trends, principles and alternatives*. Linacre Centre, London.

Lockwood, M. (ed.) (1985). *Moral dilemmas in modern medicine*. Oxford University Press, Oxford.

McMillan, R. C. Engelhardt, H. T. Jr., and Spicker, S. F. (eds.) (1987). *Euthanasia and the newborn: conflicts regarding saving lives*. D Reidel, Dordrecht.

Mason, J. K. and McCall Smith, R. A. (1983). *Law and medical ethics*. Butterworths, Sevenoaks, Kent.

Munson, R. (1979). *Intervention and reflection: basic issues in medical ethics*. Wadsworth, Belmont, CA.

Phillips, M. and Dawson, J. (1985). *Doctors' dilemmas: medical ethics and contemporary science*. Harvester Press, Brighton, Sussex.

Ramsey, P. (1978). *Ethics at the edges of life: medical and legal intersections*. Yale University Press, New Haven, CT.

Stinson, R and Stinson, P. (1983). *The long dying of Baby Andrew*. Little, Brown, Boston, MA.

US Government, President's Commission for the Study of Ethical Problems in Medicine and Biomedical and Behavioural Research (1983). *Deciding to forego life-sustaining treatment: a report on the ethical, medical and legal issues in treatment decisions*. US Government Printing Office, Washington, DC.

US National Academy of Sciences (1975). *Experiments and research with humans: values in conflict*. National Academy of Sciences, Washington, DC.

Weir, R. F. (1984). *Selective non-treatment of handicapped newborns: moral dilemmas in neonatal medicine*. Oxford University Press, Oxford.

9

Changing paediatric perceptions and perspectives

JOHN O. FORFAR

As the pattern of childhood disease changes death is no longer the expected family visitor it once was to one or more of the children of the large families of the Victorian era. Much childhood disease and disorder remain, however, to afflict, burden, and handicap, and sometimes effectively to destroy without death the lives, not only of children, but also of the adults these children become. As some diseases disappear and new ones appear, as the character of living alters, as the physical and social nature of the environment changes and means of adaptation to these changes are developed, as the World apparently becomes a much smaller place, so do perceptions of child health alter and with them child health perspectives. One characteristic of the child does not change, however, namely his basic biological make-up.

The unchanging child

The essential characteristic of the child distinguishing him from all other age groups is development; development in respect of physical growth, motor power and coordination, intellect, speech, language, the special senses, emotional control, social adaptation, and life expectation. If life is represented as the graph shown in Fig. 9.1. then paediatricians, the physicians of children, can be thought of as dealing with the left-hand side of the graph and physicians of the adult with the right. The work of the paediatrician is to promote healthy child development, to try to ensure the blossoming of all of the attributes which go to make up the normal child, and to prevent disease or other agencies from interfering with the progressive evolution of these attributes. In contrast, the work of the physician of the adult is largely concerned with holding back the processes of degeneration. Disease in the child may check developmental progress, disease in the adult is more likely to hasten degenerative processes. Childhood is the base on which adult life is built, adulthood the integrated superstructure: child health is an essential pursuit in itself but at the same time the necessary foundation for healthy adulthood. While the basic characteristics of the child change not, the responses called forth from him by the impositions of a changing world do. Paediatrics for its part has to recognize and understand these changing responses and adapt its practice and philosophy to meet them.

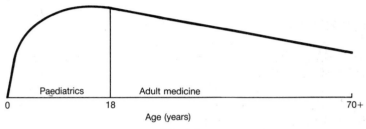

Fig. 9.1.

Old mortality and new morbidity

In 1928, the year in which the British Paediatric Association (BPA) was founded, just over 10 000 children (0–14 years) died each year per million children in Britain: sixty years earlier the corresponding number of childhood deaths was nearly 30 000. Today, 60 years *after* the founding of the BPA, the figures for childhood deaths per annum per million is just under 1000.

In 1928 there were those who considered that the improvement in childhood mortality which had taken place over the previous 60 years had been so dramatic that it was unlikely that much further improvement could be achieved: child health need be accorded little priority. Likewise there are some now who appear to be unjustifiably satisfied with a similar interpretation of today's figures. A mortality rate is a splendidly finite statistic, a measure of those children who have ceased to require any health care. It is a very inadequate measure of child health in the living. The need for paediatric services requires to be measured in terms of the number of children who survive and require help, not the number who die. Morbidity not mortality is the yardstick against which paediatric needs have to be measured. Many children who would have died in the past now survive and do so because modern medicine has saved them, but the services of modern medicine may continue to be required to sustain their health and maintain their survival.

As illustrated in Chapter 1 the fall in mortality over the past 60 years has been achieved in large measure by the ability to prevent or cure infections. The mortalities in a number of erstwhile common childhood diseases due to infection are shown in Table 1.1, p. 10. In contrast mortality from many, but not all, of the congenital disorders has altered little. Figure 9.2 shows the change in mortality in Scotland as between infections and congenital abnormalities in the 30-year period between 1945 and 1975. Congenital abnormalities are disorders present from birth, although not necessarily evident at that time. They may be of a hereditary nature (genetic) as a result of abnormal traits which can be overt or covert and present in one or both parents, due to abnormalities in the sex cell (ova/spermatozoa) union at the time of conception, or due to damage to the developing fetus *in utero* (Chapter 2). Another group of important problems is that arising from infants born too early (prematurely) or those who have suffered damage as a result of the potentially hazardous process we call birth (Chapter 3).

Short-term illness—likely cure

The control of infection has resulted from a number of factors; better nutrition of the child population, better social and environmental conditions, the introduction of preventive immunization procedures, the establishment of a force of doctors—paediatricians—and nurses who specialize in the diseases of children, and the availability of effective drugs such as antibiotics and chemotherapeutic agents. Many of the diseases due to infection are now capable of complete cure but this often depends on early and accurate diagnosis and the early application of correct treatment. To achieve these objectives a readily available and skilled primary care (general practitioner) service and a highly trained and expert hospital paediatric staff, adequate in numbers, is necessary. Thus while treatment of many childhood infections can mean a short illness and cure, delay, too few trained paediatric personnel, or, sometimes, unusual resistance of the disease itself to treatment can result in sequelae of a long-term nature, handicap, and the need for continuing medical support.

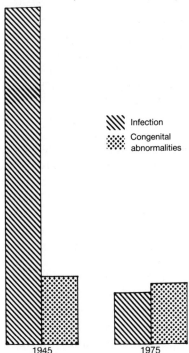

Infection

Congenital
abnormalities

1945   1975

Fig. 9.2. Relative mortalities in Scotland from infections and congenital
abnormalities in 1945 and 1975.

There are many examples of diseases which in the past were
prolonged or fatal illnesses but can now be cured, usually rapidly
(Chapter 1). Childhood tuberculosis has diminished in incidence
and changed dramatically in character as a result of public health
measures and the development of effective drug therapy. Scarlet
fever has become a rare disease as a result of apparent loss of
virulence of the causative organism, the haemolytic streptococcus,
combined with the discovery of a variety of antistreptococcal
antibiotics. Gastro-enteritis in Britain, formerly a killing disease of
infants, is now usually a mild and short-lived illness.

In a somewhat different category because it is a congenital
disorder is a threat which has in the past hung like a sword of
Damocles over many mothers throughout most of their reproductive
lives. They were threatened that their infants, unborn or not yet
conceived, might die *in utero* or just after birth due to destruction
of their blood, or survive to suffer from a severe type of jaundice,

the so-called *haemolytic disease of the new-born* (HDN) or *icterus gravis neonatorum*, which usually resulted in choreo-athetoid cerebral palsy (p. 85), deafness, or mental impairment. The fault (if such it could be called) lay in the blood groups of a husband and wife. Fifteen per cent of the population have so-called Rh negative blood and 85 per cent Rh positive blood. These are normal blood groups but where a woman is Rh negative and her husband is Rh positive (1 in 8 marriages) the pregnancy is theoretically at risk. The risk is that if the baby acquires the father's Rh positive blood group, the Rh positive blood of the baby, being 'incompatible' with the Rh negative blood group of the mother, causes 'antibodies' to develop in the mother's blood which then 'attack' and destroy the baby's blood. Far fewer pregnancies than are at theoretical risk come to harm, however, because certain subgroups within the Rh grouping and usually several pregnancies are needed to 'stimulate' the disorder.

Sixty years ago the cause of icterus gravis neonatorum was unknown. It was discovered in the early 1940s. There followed a long period of 20 years or so when techniques such as exchange transfusion of the baby at birth (replacing his blood with 'compatible' blood), intra-uterine transfusion (transfusing the fetus *in utero*), obstetric delivery of the infant before it died *in utero*, and genetic counselling of parents at risk resulted in a steady fall in mortality (Fig. 9.3). Then came the discovery in which Sir Cyril Clarke, a Past President of the Royal College of Physicians of London, played such a major part, namely that in most mothers at risk the possible adverse outcome of that risk could be prevented by administering to these mothers at delivery, or sometimes earlier, a substance (the so-called anti-D gamma-globulin) which prevented the blood group incompatibility from developing and affecting subsequent babies. The interesting biological aspect of this discovery is that the anti-D gamma-globulin used contains the very 'antibody' which causes the disease but which if administered to the mother at the appropriate time and in appropriate dosage can prevent the disease. The result of the widespread use of anti-D gamma-globulin on mortality from HDN is shown in Fig. 9.3, but these figures, reflecting only deaths, do not reveal the much larger number of surviving new-born babies who have been saved from disturbing and potentially dangerous procedures such as intra-uterine and exchange transfusion and from possible life-long deafness, mental impairment, and choreo-athetosis.

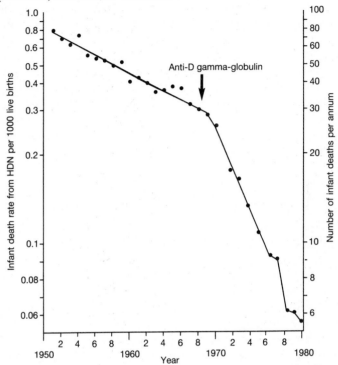

Fig. 9.3. Accelerated decline in deaths in England and Wales from Haemolytic disease of the newborn (HDN) since the introduction of prophylactic anti-D gamma globulin. Figures on the right are deaths from HDN per 100 000 live births—multiplying these figures by six gives the approximate number of actual deaths per annum in Britain. (Data supplied by Office of Population, Censuses and Surveys; graph supplied by courtesy of Sir Cyril Clarke)

Long-term illness—possible cure

In another category are the childhood diseases for which today medicine and surgery have much to offer compared with the past but at the price of prolonged, and often painful, disturbing treatment and as yet with no guarantee of cure. Examples are acute lymphatic leukaemia and serious congenital heart disease.

Thirty-five years ago the average survival time of a child who developed *acute lymphatic leukaemia* was six weeks. Treatment often merely prolonged a process of painful dying. By 1966 the average survival time of cases treated in Edinburgh had risen to one year but no case had survived more than two years. By 1976, 47 per cent were surviving ten years or more and by 1986 over 60 per cent would survive ten years or more. 'Cure' now seems a not unreasonable term to apply to many of these cases. The treatment of such children is a long process and the drugs which must be used are highly toxic with disturbing side-effects such as loss of hair (temporary) and plethora of the face. Fear of relapse is ever present. Radiation with its nauseating and depressing effects is often necessary. Family life may be disrupted in the interests of the ill child and the family is put under a severe emotional and psychological strain, not to mention financial strain, in many instances. The long-term morbidity and reduced mortality of 1988 are far more demanding on patients and medical and nursing staff and need far more resources than the short-term morbidity and high mortality of 1950. Fig. 1.8 (p. 18) indicates the improved life expectancy of the major malignant diseases of childhood.

Twenty-five years ago few infants born with *serious congenital heart disease* survived for long and there was little that could be done for them. Today the majority can be improved medically and treated surgically using techniques which require long training before they can be perfected and equipment which is expensive and demands great skill in its operation. A short-term invalidism and high mortality associated with little need for medical or nursing resources has been replaced by a morbidity which needs a great deal of both but which is now associated with hope and frequently success.

Long-term illness—palliation, symptomatic improvement, and support
For many of the hereditary and congential abnormalities cure is not yet possible. These disorders raise many of the clinical and moral dilemmas for both parents and paediatricians discussed in Chapters 2 and 4. Anxiety about the affected child is compounded by the guilt feelings which the parents may suffer on account of the genesis of their child's illness. For many such disorders, however, the therapeutic inadequacies and early deaths of yesterday have been replaced by the significantly prolonged survival and improved quality of life of today. Such a disorder is cystic fibrosis. These and other such disorders are described in Chapter 4.

Birth survival—the balance of advantage

Sixty years ago one mother died in childbirth for every 225 births; today the corresponding figures are one in every 10,000 births. Out of every 1000 infants born in 1928, 40 were still-born, 35 died in the first month of life, and another 45 died by the end of the first year: today the corresponding figures per 1000 births are 5.5 for still-births, 5.5 for first-month deaths, and 4.5 for the last eleven months of the first year. Within these figures lies one of the great dilemmas regarding the mortality/morbidity equation. Modern obstetric practice and paediatric care of the new-born infant (neonatology) ensure the survival of many infants who would have been still-born and of many who would have died shortly after birth. Further, they ensure that many infants who would have survived in the past, but would have suffered damage and disorder as a result of birth, often with permanent residual handicap, now survive in a healthy state. The dilemma arises in respect of those infants of very low birth-weight (VLBW), those who have been severely asphyxiated at birth, and those with severe congenital abnormalities who would have died in the past but now survive in a state, unfortunately, of permanent handicap due to cerebral palsy (see p. 82), mental impairment, or serious physical disorder. With the exception of obvious congenital abnormalities these infants often cannot be clearly identified from those, often apparently similarly disordered at birth, who survive in a healthy state to lead normal lives. Does neonatal intensive care enable infants who would have died to survive? Does it allow infants who would have survived but would have been permanently damaged to survive in a healthy state? Does it result in some infants who would have died surviving permanently handicapped? To the first two of these questions the answer is almost certainly in the affirmative. The answer to the third must also be in the affirmative but is hedged around with so many medical, moral, and ethical dilemmas that a simple yes or no does not do the question justice. The issues raised by the question are explored in Chapters 3 and 8.

A new disase

Textbooks of paediatrics take some time to prepare and their contents tend to reflect knowledge current up to two years before their publication date. Textbooks published as late as 1983 contained no reference to AIDS (auto-immune deficiency disease) or the virus which causes it, the human immunodeficiency virus (HIV), a virus which has an almost unique capacity to wear down inexorably the mechanisms by which the body protects itself against the microbiological threats which pervade the environment in which we live.

Whatever the moral issues surrounding AIDS, affected children are its innocent sufferers. There are two categories of affected children. A mother who acquires AIDS—most likely because she is a drug addict injecting herself intravenously with a shared needle which has been contaminated—and becomes pregnant is likely to transmit the virus to her infant. Current evidence suggests that up to two-thirds of infants born to mothers who are asymptomatic but sero-positive (i.e. as yet have developed no symptoms but have acquired the disease as shown on blood testing) will develop clinical symptoms before two years of age, symptoms which at present presage a fatal outcome. Further, there is some disputed evidence that pregnancy may activate the virus in an asymptomatic sero-positive mother producing clinical symptoms in her. From the point of view of both baby and affected mother pregnancy is to be avoided at all costs and in the present stage of knowledge should be terminated if it occurs.

The second means by which children can be affected by AIDS is through transfusion with contaminated blood. Unfortunately some children with diseases such as haemophilia, for which blood transfusion is frequently required, were infected before a test which would detect HIV contamination of blood had been developed. As the blood test does not become positive (sero-positive) until three months after initial infection it is still possible for blood obtained for transfusion during this latent period to be infected yet sero-negative (i.e. apparently uninfected).

The clinical symptoms of AIDS in childhood are recurrent infections, often of the ear, lungs, and gut, resulting in painful 'running' ears, cough with pyrexia, diarrhoea, and failure to thrive. Later, neurological symptoms with spasticity (stiffness and incoordination of muscles) usually develops.

Apart from the medical effects of AIDS the disease has enormous psychological and social implications. The state of mind of the husband who infects his wife and through her his child or of the drug-addicted teenager who becomes infected and pregnant is difficult to comprehend. AIDS has created a new dimension in apprehension, anxiety, and guilt related to promiscuity and compounded by the long 'silent' interval between a recognized incident of risk and the development of presenting symptoms. Like so many 'new' diseases, however, the fear which AIDS has generated regarding normal non-sexual contact—which constitutes very little risk—has been exaggerated. AIDS does, however, present a problem for those who have to handle specimens of blood, etc. from infected patients, those who deliver such patients in maternity units, and those who look after them in their terminal stages in intensive care units. The willing performance of these tasks by so many doctors, nurses, and technicians should be adequately recognized.

A child with haemophilia is a source of serious and constant concern to his parents, a concern aggravated by the hereditary nature of the disorder. As he grows up he is likely to be burdened with disability and anxiety. Fate dealt some such children another serious blow when it put them at risk of AIDS before the nature of this risk had been recognized and the means of obviating it discovered. Schoolchildren with AIDS are nearly all haemophiliacs infected by contaminated blood transfusion. Children at school who suffer from AIDS cause concern to the parents of other children in the school but there is no known case of a child being infected by contact in school nor even within a family where a child suffers from AIDS and other members of the family do not. As infected children may be unnecessarily stigmatized at school, knowledge that a schoolchild suffers from AIDS should be confined rigorously to the few who need to know, such as those who would care for him should he bleed. As precautionary measures in schools and elsewhere practices such as becoming 'blood brothers', ear piercing, tattooing, and sharing of toothbrushes or razors should be prohibited (DHSS 1986).

An old disorder in a new guise

Sixty years ago 'overlaying' was not uncommonly registered as a cause of death in infancy. Few would believe that overlaying is now, or was then, a common cause of infant death. These infant deaths were almost certainly 'cot deaths'. Cot death is the sudden unexpected death of an infant usually in sleep, and is not uncommon. Approximately 1400 cot deaths occur in the UK every year and cot death is now the greatest single cause of death between the ages of one month and one year in the Western World. A striking characteristic is its narrow age range, 75 per cent of cases occurring between the second and sixth months of life. Very low birth-weight increases the risk but social class does not exercise a strong influence. Subsequent siblings of infants who have suffered cot death have a higher chance of dying similarly.

Many factors have been considered to contribute to cot death but it would appear that a wide range of factors can lead to a final common end-point, namely cessation of breathing.

Unfortunately, little can be said about prevention. Good antenatal and obstetric care for the mother, avoidance of smoking, unnecessary medication during pregnancy, breast feeding, and close observation for a few days after minor illness are all steps which reduce the risk.

Understandably, cot death usually creates a family crisis. Relationships within the family may be strained by guilt, misplaced blame, and severe and persistent grief reactions. The suddenness of cot death is such that it frequently occurs when no doctor has been involved, leaving the distraught parents without the paediatric advice and support which they require under these tragic circumstances. In conjunction with the Foundation for the Study of Infant Deaths the BPA has arranged for a paediatrician with a particular interest in cot death to be available in each area to give advice and support to such bereaved parents.

Widening paediatric perspectives

The declining demands of the death-dealing diseases have allowed paediatricians to devote more attention to long-term disorders and handicap, to turn their attention more to providing care not only in the hospital but also in the community outside. Those childhood disorders, such as handicapping, behavioural, and educational disorders, which by their nature can do so much to disrupt the equanimity of family life as well as the life of the affected child, now receive much more attention. These are the disorders described in Chapter 4, plus the disorders of a psychological nature—the temper tantrums, the sleep disorders, the bed wetting, the school refusal, the hyperactivity, the stammering, the refusal to eat, the aggressive behaviour, the adolescent problems, to refer to but some of them. Specific educational difficulties often with a subtle medical basis now comprise a paediatric subspecialty. The physical, social, psychological, and environmental background against which these disorders so often occur is portrayed in Chapter 5.

Prevention, screening, and surveillance

Prevention of disease is the ultimate aim. For many diseases such as smallpox, poliomyelitis, diphtheria, tetanus, and tuberculosis specific immunization measures have been dramatically successful in prevention. Public health measures have reduced the incidence of many of the infections of the past, improved nutrition has increased resistance to many diseases.

Accidents remain a major scourge of childhood. Although road traffic instruction and seat-belts have prevented the toll of road accidents from being higher, child-proof containers have reduced the number of children poisoning themselves by swallowing medications prescribed for their parents, and swimming instruction has saved some children from drowning, 1000 children die each year from accidents on the roads or in the home, 150 000 are admitted into hospital on account of accidents and 1.5 million attend accident and emergency departments.Impressive although some of the preventive measures are and important as it is to continue striving to apply them, to improve them, and to introduce others there are unfortunately no specific preventive measures for the majority of childhood diseases.

Sixty years ago when the paediatric service in Britain was little more than embryonic, disease in childhood tended to present to the medical services late and in a much more florid form than it does today. The appreciation of illness in a child tended to depend on observing established symptoms and the gross signs of disease. Treatment often had to be directed to rescuing the child from the jaws of death and was ineffective in that it was applied too late.

As medicine advances so does it seek to recognize disease at an earlier and earlier stage in order that cure may be effective, in that it is applied early and the duration of disability reduced. Extending this concept further, medicine seeks for the same reason to *screen* for disease, to discover defects before they have revealed themselves by symptoms. Such philosophies have particular relevance in childhood. A parallel concept is that of *surveillance* whereby a child with any recognized departure from normal is kept under review on a continuing basis so that necessary supportive steps may be foreseen and remedial measures taken should there be any evidence of incipient deterioration.

Routine screening is now widely practised in respect of new-born infants born in hospital—and very few births in Britain take place outside hospital. New-born babies are examined once or twice before discharge from the maternity hospital in which they are born for any detectable defect such as congenital heart disease, cleft palate, or abnormal abdominal organs. In addition certain specific procedures are usually carried out.

Congenital dislocation of the hip (CDH)

One of the special screening procedures is for congenital dislocation of the hip, a disorder present in one in 250 infants and one which, if untreated, will make walking difficult and abnormal later in childhood, and later still is likely to result in osteo-arthritis of the hip joint. Treatment in the past was usually instituted when the disorder revealed itself after one or two years and usually consisted of surgical operation on the hip joint, a procedure not always successful. Screening of the new-born infant using a simple clinical test and confirmation of the abnormality by radiology or ultrasound now reveals most cases and enables successful and simple treatment by a splinting technique to be applied on an out-patient basis.

Phenylketonuria (PKU) and hypothyroidism (cretinism)

Another type of neonatal screening procedure is the metabolic screening test (metabolic refers to biochemical change involving living tissue). Two such tests are commonly applied with a view to recognizing phenylketonuria (PKU) and hypothyroidism. *Phenylketonuria* is an inborn biochemical abnormality which within a few weeks of birth will render a child irretrievably mentally defective. The damage is done long before the mental defect can be recognized on the basis of ordinary clinical examination—by that time it is too late. Yet the damage can be prevented if it is recognized within a few days of birth that the disease is present. Such recognition is only possible by screening all babies at birth using a biochemical test on a few drops of the baby's blood. Thereafter, throughout childhood and adolescence at least, a highly specialized diet is necessary to keep the disease at bay and to allow an affected child to develop normally, physically, and intellectually. Leaving humanitarian issues aside, the cost of screening all children so as to detect the 1 in 8000 who suffer from this disease is far less than the cost of caring for one mentally impaired child throughout childhood into adult life.

Hypothyroidism, or cretinism as it is more commonly known in lay parlance, is a traditional cause of imbecility. It occurs in approximately 1 in 6000 infants and, if not recognized until the gross features of the disease are manifest, irreversible mental impairment is likely. A routine metabolic test applied a few days after birth reveals the condition, which is due to deficient functioning of the thyroid gland. Recognition allows replacement treatment (oral), which is usually successful, to be instituted.

Other 'screenable' disorders

CDH, PKU, and hypothyroidism are but three examples where screening tests confer great benefit on the infant screened. There are others, less dramatic. Screening tests are available for tuberculosis, previous infection with German measles (important for women in the child-bearing period), hidden urinary tract infection, high blood pressure, etc.

Certain other screening tests raise controversial issues. *Thalassaemia* and *sickle cell disease* are two very common blood diseases in certain parts of the world, particularly Africa. They can exist in the major (homozygous) form or the minor (heterozygous or carrier) form. The minor forms may not even reveal themselves without screening. The offspring of two individuals each of whom may have the minor form has a high chance of suffering from the major form. Thus screening can play an important part in marriage and genetic counselling but such screening programmes in communities at risk have sometimes been misunderstood and in some communities have been considered by those revealed as carriers as a form of victimization. Yet a third possible role of screening is the protection of the public as has been mooted under certain circumstances for AIDS.

Parental and public perceptions of responsibilities to children and attitudes to their health

The birth rate per 1000 population is today approximately 13; a century ago it was nearly three-times that. There are fewer children today than there used to be and a crude corollary of this is that children have now acquired a scarcity value which they did not formerly possess. As the repositories of all their parents' hopes and ambitions, more is expected of the one or two children who constitute the present-day family.

Family disruption and family disadvantage

In striking contrast to parental expectations regarding their children is parental responsibility towards their children in respect of their own marriage status. The concept of the prototype family, the so called nuclear family of two parents—the father working—and two children, becomes increasingly irrelevant in the light of one marriage in three now ending in divorce (175 000 divorces per annum) and one child in eight living in a one-parent family (a million single-parent families). The appropriateness of 'keeping the family together for the sake of the children' is a subject of some debate but it is not an idea which seems to commend itself to many parents today or receive much consideration as they thrash out their own personal objections to their marriage partners.

Poor physical development, ill health, less satisfactory behaviour patterns, and inadequate school attainments, along with poor parental interest in their children's education, are commoner in children who come from homes which are disadvantaged as judged by low income (on supplementary benefit or receiving free school meals), large families (five or more children), single-parent families, or poor housing (more than 1.5 persons per room) (Wedge and Prosser 1973). The unanswered question is the relationship between the perceived environmental disadvantages and the child's development and performance. Are the environmental disadvantages the cause of the child's poor performance or is it that unsatisfactory intrinsic attributes in parents who are themselves poor performers are transmitted genetically to their children so that they too perform poorly? Both sets of factors are likely to contribute but the onus on society is to ameliorate or remove as best it can the disadvantaging environmental factors which it has the power to control. The divorce rated in unemployed men is twice the national average.

Media violence

The media, particularly in the form of television and video, have brought to many homes the opportunity for children to see physical violence, sexual violence, and obscenity. The World, so often, is presented as a violent and alarming place. It is difficult to exclude children from parental viewing and many parents see no obligation to do so. Barlow and Hill (1985) found that one-third of children aged 7 to 8 years and over 50 per cent of children aged 15 to 16 years had seen one or more obscene videos. Ninety per cent of paediatricians consider that video 'nasties' are sometimes harmful to children and 17 per cent believe that they are always harmful. Acute symptoms recognized to be associated with video nasties are nightmares, sleeplessness, bed wetting, fears and anxieties about being left alone (Gray 1987). Often the degree of violence portrayed is such that anyone with any knowledge of the frailty of the human frame would recognize that such violence would almost certainly result in serious or fatal injury. Yet the assaulted victim of the television screen so often gets up, dusts himself down, and carries on with a nonchalant shake of the head. How many tragic and unintended results of violence are due to misguided media-induced assumptions regarding the degree of trauma which the human body can sustain?

Expectations of medicine

Influenced by the dramatic, highly selected and often un-representative successes of medicine which the media so often present, parental expectations of medicine are often higher than are justified. Successes achieved in some areas of medicine are not necessarily matched in all and the assumption that they are can lead to great parental disappointment and frustration. Allied to that, parents often experience guilt feelings when their children are ill. A few rationalize their frustration and guilt in the form of antagonism to doctors and nurses caring for their children. Paediatricians understand this, less experienced doctors and nurses may not always do so. Balancing that to some extent is the greater knowledge of the public about medical matters and their desire for information.

Parent–hospital relationships

Most parents rightly wish for explanations, of the steps taken to diagnose and manage their child's illnesses, of the purpose of any procedures carried out, of the rationale of any programme of care proposed, and of likely outcome and future prospects. The great majority of paediatricians consider that discussion of such matters with parents is an important part of managing any child's illness.

The important role of parents in all aspects of their children's health and welfare is universally recognized by paediatricians. Parents are their children's nurses, their children's supporters, their children's advisers and persuaders, *par excellence*. Paediatricians and the paediatric service supply the professional knowledge, the expertise, the technology which the parents themselves cannot supply. Paediatricians today regard parents as their co-partners and seek parental involvement, whenever possible, in the management of children in hospital: they recognize the important part parents play in assisting an ill child's recovery. How different the position was 60 years ago when hospital doctors tended to assume exclusive authority for children under their care. Parental visitations to hospital wards were looked upon as something of a nuisance to be restricted to one hour once or twice a week. Sometimes parents were excluded from the hospital for the first week of a child's admission on the assumption (very false as we now know) that this would enable the child to become 'acclimatized to the hospital'.

Most paediatric departments, but regretably not all hospital departments admitting children, recognize the importance of ensuring that parents have free access to their children when the latter are in hospital (Plates IX, X, and XVI). They go further, and seek admission for the mother when a child is admitted to hospital. Not all hospitals, however, have accommodation available for such a purpose. Given the need, few mothers stand on ceremony and many a floor mattress, easy chair, or imported camp-bed is pressed into service in providing overnight accommodation for mothers. Chapter 7 presents a graphic account of some of the changes which have taken place in children's hospital wards over the past few decades.

The changing child health service

Paediatricians

When the BPA was established in 1928 its original membership was 56; today its membership exceeds 2000. In 1928 paediatric practice in Britain lagged far behind that in the USA and some of the European countries. Dr Donald Paterson, a Canadian who had qualified in Edinburgh and was on the staff of the Hospital for

Sick Children, Great Ormond Street, London was the prime mover in recognizing the need for the formation of the BPA.

The development of the National Health Service
One effect of war is to draw attention to the health of young men and by implication, to the health of children. Concern at the poor health of young men examined for service in the Boer War led to the establishment of the School Health Service in 1908. After the First World War the Child Welfare Service was established, in 1918, and after the Second World War, the National Health Service (NHS), from which children were major beneficiaries, was established in 1948.

The establishment of the NHS represented two major advances in child health practice. Prior to the NHS there were few doctors who practiced paediatrics wholly because, in the voluntary hospitals which provided the major part of the hospital service, consultants were unpaid for their services and had to rely on private practice for their incomes. Impecunious parents were often unable to afford private consultant fees so that consultant practice tended to be concentrated on wealthier adults with the deployment of a disproportionate number of the most highly qualified members of the medical profession and of medical resources to that group. Nor were children covered by the National Insurance Acts so that the provision of general practitioner care for their children could constitute a serious financial burden for parents. Those who worked in the hospital service before the inception of the NHS remember the mass of children and parents who attended the children's out-patient departments of the voluntary hospitals on Saturday mornings and on public holidays because at these times father, who attended or stayed at home to look after the other children, would not lose a day's pay by so doing (Plate III). One of the great and lasting achievements of the NHS is that it changed all that. Hospital consultants, paid for their services, could now specialize in the diseases of children without suffering the severe financial disadvantage previously associated with that type of practice. Whatever the merits of private medical care for the adult those who remember the gross inadequacies of the medical care of children in the pre-NHS days or, no matter how conservative their political views, see the continuing inadequacy of much of the new generation of private hospital facilities for children, would be likely to view with apprehension any return to a system in which private medicine formed any major part of the hospital care of children.

The second major advance of the NHS was that it also ensured that every child could have a general practitioner as a primary care physician.

In parallel with the establishment of the NHS more and more of the universities began to recognize their responsibilities for providing more adequate teaching and research in child health. Although a few universities had established Chairs in Child Health earlier (Edinburgh had done so in 1931) the majority of such chairs were established in the post-war era.

The need for an integrated child health service

The NHS at its establishment did not incorporate the School Health Service and the Child Welfare Service, both of which continued to be run, as they had been previously, by local authorities. In view of the changes effected by the introduction of the NHS the continued tripartite arrangement of hospital, general practitioner, and local authority child health services was a mistake.

The local authority element of the service became increasingly isolated from the mainstream of paediatrics. The doctors in it certainly had expertise in assessing developmental progress and in immunization but their lack of contact with the wider field of paediatrics, the absence of appropriate postgraduate training opportunities for them, and the increasing provision by general practitioners of the services which in the pre-NHS days had been provided by local authority doctors diminished the role and significance of the local authority service. The incorporation of the local authority child health services into the NHS in 1974 without any change in the role and deployment of the doctors in them did little to resolve the problem.

The need to integrate the child health services was recognized in the Brotherston Report (1973) and in the Court Report (1976) but the implementation of these has been delayed by the difficulties in incorporating that element of the service formerly provided by local authorities—now called the Community Child Health Service—into the hospital (secondary care) and general practice (primary care) elements of the service. Now it would appear that agreement on integration is close and it is hoped that government will take the steps necessary to implement this agreement. The primary care service will be based on general practice with general practitioners progressively increasing their participation in preventive practice as well as the curative health care which until now has been their main preoccupation. Community health doctors will work, where appropriate, with general practitioners, or where the provision of general practitioner based community child health services is inadequate will continue to provide such on their own. Consultant paediatricians, inappropriately described for so long as confining themselves to hospitals whereas much of the work of many lay in community services, will be responsible for the secondary care service and more of them will work primarily in the community as consultant paediatricians with a special interest in community child health.

These new arrangements imply different yardsticks of measurement of work and 'productivity'. The success and efficiency of a child health service and the resources made available to it should not be measured in terms of hospital beds. Paediatricians wish to keep children out of hospital beds as far as possible, believing as they do that children are best cared for at home when that is practicable and that the disturbing experience of hospital admission should be avoided except for those for whom admission is essential. Given adequate resources more children could be seen as out-patients rather than be admitted to hospital. Out-patient services which reduce in-patient admissions represent an economy.

The need to concentrate child health services

In an earlier era when paediatric care often represented little more than extended mothering it was appropriate for children to be cared for in small local hospitals, even cottage hospitals, provided they were not in adult wards subject to the sights and sounds in such, to which children should not be exposed. Today the position is different. The role of the children's hospital or paediatric department of a general hospital is to effect the early diagnosis of disease and to provide those forms of treatment which cannot be provided at home. Modern diagnosis is increasingly accurate and modern treatment increasingly effective, but they are so in terms of greater professional expertise and specialization among paediatricians and children's nurses and the availability of modern technical resources which are increasingly expensive and complex. Such expertise and resources have to be concentrated; they cannot be provided everywhere because of the highly trained professional and technical staff necessary to operate them and because of the cost. The inevitable and unfortunate corollary of this necessary concentration is that children now have to travel further for any hospital-based services which they require. Those who for partisan or political purposes demand the retention of small paediatric units in towns or villages which cannot justify proper units do children no service. Parents given the choice of the best paediatric service at a distance or an inferior one close at hand nearly always opt appropriately for the best service. The need is that the additional burden imposed on them by repeated travelling to a centralized department should be recognized and where necessary the financial burden of the travelling mitigated. The scattering of small-sized children's hospitals or units by dispersing and diluting resources can mean that the central units are deprived of the resources and staff which they require. They are an important factor in the excessive hours which doctors have to work in acute hospital departments, such as paediatric departments, because so often they make it impossible for the advised one night on duty in three rota to be implemented. A necessary concomitant of more centralized hospital departments for children is that children's out-patient and community services should be strengthened (Scottish Home and Health Department 1984, 1985).

The changing pattern of hospital admissions for children

Somewhat paradoxically, despite the desire of paediatricians, of parents, and, where they can be asked, of children to avoid hospital admission the number of children admitted to hospital is increasing not falling. The rise in England and Wales per 1000 population aged 14 years or under was from 22.3 to 38.6 in the ten years from 1974 to 1984. There are probably three reasons for this.

First children's hospitals and departments have changed their role. One of the conclusions reached by the assessors of the health service in Scotland before the introduction of the NHS was that there were too few beds to meet the demand for hospital beds for children who were acutely ill. The former role of the children's hospital or department was to admit children who 'were so ill that they had to be admitted into hospital' and so ill, too, that they could justify taking up one of the scarce beds. Such seriously ill children were often admitted into hospital too late; late diagnosis reduced their chance of survival or meant a prolonged illness with